CARDIOVASCULAR BENEFITS OF OMEGA-3 POLYUNSATURATED FATTY ACIDS

Solvay Pharmaceuticals Conferences

Series Editors

Werner Cautreels, Claus Steinborn and Lechoslaw Turski

Volume 7

Previously published in this series

ISSN 1566-7685

Cardiovascular Benefits of Omega-3 Polyunsaturated Fatty Acids

Edited by

B. Maisch

Philipps University of Marburg, Marburg, Germany

and

R. Oelze

Solvay Pharmaceuticals, Hannover, Germany

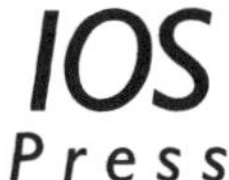

IOS
Press

Amsterdam • Berlin • Oxford • Tokyo • Washington, DC

ISBN 978-1-58603-707-9
Library of Congress Control Number: 2006939183

Publisher
IOS Press
Nieuwe Hemweg 6B
1013 BG Amsterdam
Netherlands
fax: +31 20 687 0019
e-mail: order@iospress.nl

Distributor in the UK and Ireland
Gazelle Books Services Ltd.
White Cross Mills
Hightown
Lancaster LA1 4XS
United Kingdom
fax: +44 1524 63232
e-mail: sales@gazellebooks.co.uk

Distributor in the USA and Canada
IOS Press, Inc.
4502 Rachael Manor Drive
Fairfax, VA 22032
USA
fax: +1 703 323 3668
e-mail: iosbooks@iospress.com

Cardiovascular Benefits of Omega-3 Polyunsaturated Fatty Acids
B. Maisch and R. Oelze (Eds.)
IOS Press, 2006

Preface

**"The Solvay Pharmaceutical Conferences:
where industry meets academia in a search for novel therapies"**

Therapy for Sudden Death Still Awaited

During the last decades progress has been made in the treatment of patients who survived myocardial infarction. The implementation of coronary care units and evolution of public education to encourage rapid response, development of catheter-based revascularization techniques, greater emphasis on cardiac rehabilitation, and improved therapy have contributed to improvement of prognosis for patients with myocardial infarction. The introduction of aspirin, thrombolytics, ß-blockers, ACE-inhibitors and statins led to reduction in both short-term and immediate mortality rates among patients suffering from myocardial infarction. Nevertheless, patients who survive an acute myocardial infarction are at high risk, with life expectancy half that of their peers who have not experienced similar events, and with increased risk for subsequent cardiovascular events and death. The risk of sudden death increases with severity of systolic dysfunction after myocardial infarction. Sudden death has proved to be more difficult to treat than coronary disease.

In recent years, it has become clear that in addition to risk factors such as overweight, lack of exercise, smoking, hypertension and hypercholesterolemia, psychosocial factors play a key role for prognosis in patients with myocardial infarction. Depression, anxiety, perceived social support and social desirability may have an effect on mortality and morbidity in such patients. Therefore, there is high medical need for drugs which lower the incidence of sudden death and have an effect on other risk factors such as depression.

A pharmaceutical preparation of highly purified and concentrated Ω-3 polyunsaturated acids, OMACOR®, may represent such a drug. It lowers the incidence of sudden death in patients with myocardial infarction and decreases depression.

This volume summarizes lectures delivered during the symposium entitled "Effect of Ω-3 polyunsaturated fatty acids on different risk factors in patients with cardiovascular disease" presented during the European Cardiology Society Congress in Stockholm (Sweden) in 2005. In addition, aspects of prevention of cardiovascular disease, risk factors, and pharmacokinetics of Ω-3 fatty acids ethyl esters have been considered.

W. Cautreels
C. Steinborn
L. Turski

List of Contributors

Alter, P.
Molecular Cardiology Laboratory, Department of Internal Medicine and Cardiology, Philipps University of Marburg, Karl-von-Frisch-Strasse 1, D-35033 Marburg, Germany

Annemans, L.
HEDM-IMS, Rue De Crayer 6, 1000 Brussels, Belgium
Ghent University, Sint-Pietersnieuwstraat 25, 9000 Ghent, Belgium

Cautreels, W.
Solvay Pharmaceuticals, Brussels, Belgium

Connolly, S.J
Faculty of Health Sciences, McMaster University, 237 Barton Street E., Hamilton, Ontario L8L 2X2, Canada

Frasure-Smith, N.
Centre Hospitalier de l'Université de Montréal, Hôpital Notre-Dame, Recherche Psychiatrie, Pavillon L-C Simard, 1560 rue Sherbrooke Est, Montréal, Québec, Canada H2L 4M1

Healey, J.S.
Faculty of Health Sciences, McMaster University, 237 Barton Street E., Hamilton, Ontario L8L 2X2, Canada

Huber, G.
1st Medical Department, SMZ-Ost/Danube Hospital, Langobardenstrasse 122, A-1220 Vienna, Austria

Kawalec, P.
HTA Center, Nuszkiewicza Street 13/19, Krakow, Poland
Institute of Public Health, Collegium Medium, Jagiellonian University, Grzegorzecka Street 20, Krakow, Poland

Lamotte, M.
HEDM-IMS, Rue De Crayer 6, 1000 Brussels, Belgium

Lespérance, F.
Centre Hospitalier de l'Université de Montréal, Hôpital Notre-Dame, Recherche Psychiatrie, Pavillon L-C Simard, 1560 rue Sherbrooke Est, Montréal, Québec, Canada H2L 4M1

Maisch, B.
Molecular Cardiology Laboratory, Department of Internal Medicine and Cardiology, Philipps University of Marburg, Baldingerstrasse, D-35043 Marburg, Germany

Rupp, H.
Molecular Cardiology Laboratory, Department of Internal Medicine and Cardiology, Philipps University of Marburg, Karl-von-Frisch-Strasse 1, D-35033 Marburg, Germany

Rupp, T.P.
Molecular Cardiology Laboratory, Department of Internal Medicine and Cardiology, Philipps University of Marburg, Karl-von-Frisch-Strasse 1, D-35033 Marburg, Germany

Selimi, D.
1st Medical Department, SMZ-Ost/Danube Hospital, Langobardenstrasse 122, A-1220 Vienna, Austria

Severus, W.E.
Ludwig-Maximilians-University, Department of Psychiatry, Nußbaumstrasse 7, 80336 Munich, Germany

Steinborn, C.
Solvay Pharmaceuticals, Hannover, Germany

Turski, L.
Solvay Pharmaceuticals, Weesp, The Netherlands

Verboom, C.N.
Solvay Pharmaceuticals, Hannover, Germany

Vik, H.
Pronova Biocare, P.O. Box 420, N-1327 Lysaker, Norway

Vinereanu, D.
University of Medicine and Pharmacy Carol Davila, Cardiology, University Hospital of Bucharest, Splaiul Independentei 169, Bucharest, 05098, Romania

Wagner, D.
Molecular Cardiology Laboratory, Department of Internal Medicine and Cardiology, Philipps University of Marburg, Karl-von-Frisch-Strasse 1, D-35033 Marburg, Germany

Weber, H.S.
1st Medical Department, SMZ-Ost/Danube Hospital, Langobardenstrasse 122, A-1220 Vienna, Austria

Zoellner, Y.
Solvay Pharmaceuticals GmbH, Global Health Economics, P.O. Box 220, D-30002 Hannover, Germany

Contents

Conference Preface

and

Keynote Lecture

3

Conference Preface

Omega-3 Polyunsaturated Fatty Acids: When Nature Writes the Draft to Evidence-Based Medicine

It still happens that nature writes the draft for a fundamental contribution to medical textbooks: such a classic example is the observation that Greenland Eskimos eating a diet high in omega-3 polyunsaturated fatty acids (PUFAs) from fish and sea mammals [1,2] had an unexpectedly low cardiac mortality.

Coming from such observational evidence, the next logical step in medical research is to go to evidence-based medicine or truly to the heart of the matter: the US Physicians' Health Study [3] demonstrated in the 4th quartile of enroled individuals a 50% reduction of sudden cardiac death, if at least one fish meal per day was consumed. Three randomized trials demonstrated a reduction in the risk of sudden death by dietary changes and supplementation of the daily diet increasing omega-3 PUFA intake [4-6]. GISSI-Prevenzione [6] has been the landmark trial with 11324 patients enroled to show a reduction of sudden cardiac death by 45% in post-myocardial infarction patients, which was attributed to the EPA and DHA ethyl esters.

In addition, Mozaffarian *et al* [7] analysed the risk of 5201 men and women older than 65 years from the Medicare eligibility list and found that consumption of tuna or broiled or baked fish was associated with a lower incidence of atrial fibrillation. Similarly, Calo *et al* [8] reported a reduction of postoperative atrial fibrillation by 54.4% in 160 randomized patients after CABG.

As pointed out by **Weber** *et al* in their contribution to this book [9], this clear evidence was reflected in the European Society of Cardiology guidelines for the prevention of sudden death [10,11]: omega-3 fatty acids (EPA & DHA) were rated as a class IIa, level of evidence B recommendation for the secondary prevention of sudden death after myocardial infarction. Remarkably, the relative risk reduction (RR) for <u>total</u> mortality was 0.7 for EPA/DHA, 0.83 for ACE-inhibitors and 0.77 for beta-blockers. For sudden cardiac death it was an impressive relative risk reduction of 0.55 for EPA/DHA, whereas it was only 0.8 for ACE-inhibitors and 0.74 for beta-blockers.

Rupp *et al* [12] established a gaschromatic micromethod for analyzing EPA and DHA levels on a routine basis and could show that the supplementation of 1 g/day of highly purified EPA and DHA ethyl esters (OMACOR®) increased EPA from 0.6 to 1.4% and DHA from 2.9 to 4.3%. He suggests, also in his book-chapter, an EPA/arachidonic acid ratio as diagnostic parameter for the identification and reduction of pro-inflammatory eicosanoids and cytokines and recommends 1 g/day of EPA and DHA in CAD patients to reach the level of n-PUFAs in the GISSI-Prevention study, which prevented sudden cardiac death.

Atherosclerosis is the leading cause of death worldwide. 3.8 million men and 3.4 million women die each year from coronary artery disease alone. In Germany, death by cardiovascular disease has for the last three decades accounted for roughly 50% of all deaths, more than twice the incidence of neoplastic disease. Cardiovascular disease accounts for 11.8% in men and 10.5% in women of all disability-adjusted life-years lost. But as pointed out by **Vinereanu** in his contribution to this book [13], the age and gender standardised trends in cardiovascular mortality show different directions in Europe: whereas cardiovascular morbity and mortality are still increasing in Eastern Europe they are decreasing in Western Europe and in the USA. This decrease in Western Europe occurs despite the alarming increase of diabetes, metabolic syndrome and overweight even in adolescents. Overall in the worldwide survey of people aged 15-59 years, coronary artery disease is already the second largest group of deaths. Major risk factors for atherosclerosis have been clearly identified in the last century and categorized as conventional and new risk factors. Their number has been increasing ever since the beginning of the Framingham Heart Study in 1948. Remarkably, the hierarchy of risk factors for different types of atherosclerotic diseases was best evaluated in the INTERHEART study. By multivariate analysis, current smoking and a raised ApoB/ApoA1 ratio were the strongest risk factors, followed by a history of diabetes, hypertension, and psychosocial factors. Lifestyle modifications which are beneficial are the daily consumption of fruits or vegetables and regular physical activity.

In carotid atherosclerosis, which is responsible of more than 20% of all strokes in the Framingham Heart Study, the most powerful risk factors were age followed by smoking, hypertension, and raised blood lipids. For peripheral arterial atherosclerotic disease, hypertension, smoking, and diabetes are the most important risk factors.

The preventive benefit of n-3 PUFAs in patients with coronary artery disease has historically been attributed to direct interference with lipid metabolism. Presently we know much better, that it is hardly this influence on cholesterol, LDL and HDL-levels but the benefit comes from more complicated and more specific modes of action: **Rupp and coworkers** summarize in their contribution [14] the pathophysiological and pharmacological basis for interfering of n-3 PUFAs with the electrical instability of the remodelled or ischaemic heart. It has been shown by Xiao and Leaf [15] that the free fatty acids of EPA and DHA but not other fatty acids inhibit the Na^+ channel activity which occurs rapidly and can be washed out. In addition, the cardiac Na^+-Ca^{2+} exchanger [16] and the L-type Ca^{2+} channel [17], which has been inferred particularly in after-depolarisations, were inhibited. Further clinical support for anti-arrhythmogenic effects of omega-3 fatty acids was provided in the study of Calo *et al* [8].

But pathophysiologically coherent conclusions may not always be so coherent in everyday reality. Three recently published smaller ICD trials, in a situation different from acute post-MI situation in GISSI-Prevenzione, examined patients who had a defibrillator implanted for the incidence of arrhythmic events. Raitt *et al* [18], in a possibly underpowered study of 200 randomized patients, could not demonstrate a reduction of incidences of ventricular tachycardia and only a trend for less episodes of ventricular fibrillation. Leaf *et al* [19] could show in a secondary outcome analysis that fish oil prevented ventricular arrhythmic events more effectively than olive oil but missed this point in the primary outcome analysis. The SOFA-trial by Brouwer *et al* [20], when comparing fish oil vs. placebo in a similar ICD setting with 273 patients, only showed a trend but not a significant benefit. Remarkably, Burr *et al* (2003) in recent study examining the effect of the advice to increase fish oil consumption in patients with angina, showed a lack of benefit under these circumstances [5]. All these latter quasi-neutral studies share the following common deficiencies: they lack the measurement of EPA and DHA in the trial population. So in the case of the last mentioned study by Burr *et al.* [5] we do not know whether patients really followed the advice to increase fish oil consumption or not, since compliance was not measured. And in the 3 ICD studies one should be aware of the fact that they involved only 4 percent of the study population of the GISSI-Prevention trial in a situation not analogous to the acute post-MI situation. For this reason they may be considered as "convenience" trials. Rupp *et al* [12,14] hypothesize that this may be due to the fact that in acute infarction free EPA and DHA are raised in advance to levels required for their anti-arrhythmogenic action by the event and sympathetic drive, whereas the ICD is expected to terminate re-entrant ventricular tachycardias or ventricular fibrillation before a marked sympathetic activation and release of EPA and DHA occurs.

An additional intriguing possibility is the observation that the process of adverse dilatation of the heart could be attenuated by EPA and DHA as shown in the pressure overloaded rat heart.

Connolly and Healy [21], when reviewing the data on the protective effect of n-3 PUFAs on cardiovascular deaths in their chapter, underline the recommendations of the American Heart Association and the European Society of Cardiology and come to the conclusion that the benefit of secondary and probably also of primary prevention by n-3 PUFAs is based primarily on avoiding episodes of sudden cardiac death. That the costs for secondary prevention after acute myocardial infarction by n-3 PUFAs are well worthwhile and can be calculated in life-years gained (LYG) as the price to be paid is pointed out by **Lamotte, Annemans, Kawalec and Zoellner** in their chapter [22] on the socio-economic impact of this treatment. But the society must be willing to pay a threshold of about 20 000 EUR/LYG.

The **OMACOR authors** in this book [23] describe the avenue of newly planned and carried out clinical trials to expand the spectrum of application of EPA and DHA: ASCEND will evaluate serious (cardio)vascular events in a randomized clinical trial (RCT) which is four-armed and enroles 10 000 patients with diabetes mellitus. Treatment options are OMACOR® 1 g/day both in combination with 100 mg aspirin and without vs. placebo. AFORRD is also directed to type-2 diabetes patients but in a dose of 2 g/day.

Beyond the effect on coronary artery disease and sudden cardiac death omega-3 supplementation has a clearly warranted effect on the reduction of post-infarction depression and, remarkably, also on depressive patients not suffering from CAD, as shown by **Frasure-Smith and Lespérance** in their own scientific work [24] represented here and by **Severus** in his overview on depression and n-3 PUFAs in this book [25]. These interesting data may expand the therapeutic spectrum of OMACOR® considerably in the near future.

In summary, this book on omega-3 fatty acids gives an up to date reappraisal for the use of n-3 PUFAs in different fields of medicine. It has been both a privilege and a distinct pleasure to orchestrate the authors in this "concert" of various but related topics.

Bernhard Maisch

References

[1]   H.O. Bang, J. Dyerberg, A.B. Nielsen. Plasma lipid and lipoprotein pattern in Greenlandic West-coast Eskimos. *Lancet* **1** (1971) 1143-1145.
[2]   N. Kromann and A. Green. Epidemiological studies in the Upernavik district, Greenland. Incidence of some chronic diseases 1950-1974. *Acta Med. Scand.* **208** (1980) 401-406.

[3]   C.M. Albert, C.H. Hennekens, C.J. O'Donnell *et al.* Fish consumption and risk of sudden cardiac death. The US Physicians' Health Study. *JAMA* **279** (1998) 23-28.

[4]   M. de Lorgeril, S. Renaud, N. Mamelle *et al.* Mediterranean alpha-linolenic acid-rich diet in secondary prevention of coronary heart disease. *Lancet* **343** (1994) 1454-1459.

[5]   M.L. Burr, A.M. Fehily, J.F. Gilbert *et al.* Effects of changes in fat, fish, and fibre intakes on death and myocardial reinfarction: diet and reinfarction trial (DART). *Lancet* **2** (1989) 757-761.

[6]   R. Marchioli, F. Barzi, E. Bomba *et al.* Early protection against sudden death by n-3 polyunsaturated fatty acids after myocardial infarction: time-course analysis of the results of the Gruppo Italiano per lo Studio della Sopravvivenza nell'Infarto Miocardico (GISSI)-Prevenzione. *Circulation* **105** (2002) 1897-1903.

[7]   D. Mozaffarian, B.M. Psaty, E.B. Rimm *et al.* Fish intake and risk of incident atrial fibrillation. *Circulation* **110** (2004) 368-373.

[8]   L. Calo, L. Bianconi, F. Colivicchi *et al.* N-3 fatty acids for the prevention of atrial fibrillation after coronary artery bypass surgery: a randomized, controlled trial. *J. Am. Coll. Cardiol.* **45** (2005) 1723-1728.

[9]   H. Weber, D. Selimi, G. Huber. Prevention of cardiovascular diseases and highly concentrated n-3 polyunsaturated fatty acids (PUFAs) (2006). *In this book, chapter 4.*

[10]   S.G. Priori, E. Aliot, C. Blomstrom-Lundqvist *et al.* Task force on sudden cardiac death of the European Society of Cardiology. *Eur. Heart J.* **22** (2001) 1374-1450.

[11]   S.G. Priori, E. Aliot, C. Blomstrom-Lundqvist *et al.* Update of the guidelines on sudden cardiac death of the European Society of Cardiology. *Eur. Heart J.* **24** (2003) 13-15.

[12]   H. Rupp, D. Wagner, T. Rupp *et al.* Risk stratification by the "EPA+DHA Level" and the "EPA/AA ratio" focus on anti-inflammatory and antiarrhythmogenic effects of long-chain omega-3 fatty acids. *Herz* **29** (2004) 673-685.

[13]   D. Vinereanu. Risk factors for atherosclerotic disease: present and future (2006). *In this book, chapter 1.*

[14]   H. Rupp, T.P. Rupp, D. Wagern *et al.* Microdetermination of fatty acids by gas chromatography and cardiovascular risk stratification by the "EPA+DEHA level" (2006). *In this book, chapter 2.*

[15]   Y.F. Xiao, J.X. Kang, J.P. Morgan *et al.* Blocking effects of polyunsaturated fatty acids on Na^+ channels of neonatal rat ventricular myocytes. *Proc. Natl. Acad. Sci. U.S.A.* **92** (1995) 11000-11004.

[16]   Y.F. Xiao, Q. Ke, Y. Chen *et al.* Inhibitory effect of n-3 fish oil fatty acids on cardiac Na^+/Ca^{2+} exchange currents in HEK293t cells. *Biochem. Biophys. Res. Commun.* **321** (2004) 116-123.

[17]   Y.F. Xiao, A.M. Gomez, J.P. Morgan *et al.* Suppression of voltage-gated L-type Ca^{2+} currents by polyunsaturated fatty acids in adult and neonatal rat ventricular myocytes. *Proc. Natl. Acad. Sci. U.S.A.* **94** (1997) 4182-4187.

[18]   M.H. Raitt, W.E. Connor, C. Morris *et al.* Fish oil supplementation and risk of ventricular tachycardia and ventricular fibrillation in patients with implantable defibrillators: a randomized controlled trial. *JAMA* **293** (2005) 2884-2891.

[19]   A. Leaf, C.M. Albert, M. Josephson *et al.* Prevention of fatal arrhythmias in high-risk subjects by fish oil n-3 fatty acid intake. *Circulation* **112** (2005) 2762-2768.

[20]   I.A. Brouwer, P.L. Zock, A.J. Camm *et al.* Effect of fish oil on ventricular tachyarrhythmia and death in patients with implantable cardioverter defibrillators: the Study on Omega-3 Fatty Acids and Ventricular Arrhythmia (SOFA) randomized trial. *JAMA* **295** (2006) 2613-2619.

[21]   S.J. Connolly and J.S. Healey. Omega-3 fatty acids and sudden arrhythmic death (2006). *In this book, chapter 5.*

[22]   M. Lamotte, L. Annemans, P. Kawalec *et al.* A multi-country health economic evaluation of highly concentrated n-3 polyunsaturated fatty acids (PUFAs) in the secondary prevention after myocardial infraction (MI) (2006). *In this book, chapter 8.*

[23]   OMACOR-authors. OMACOR® in clinical development: a survey of current trials (2006). *In this book, chapter 9.*

[24]   N. Frasure-Smith and F. Lespérance. Depression and coronary artery disease: epidemiology and potential mechanisms (2006). *In this book, chapter 6.*

[25]   W.E. Severus. Effects of omega - 3 polyunsaturated fatty acids on depression (2006). *In this book, chapter 7.*

Cardiovascular Benefits of Omega-3 Polyunsaturated Fatty Acids
B. Maisch and R. Oelze (Eds.)
IOS Press, 2006

Risk Factors for Atherosclerotic Disease: Present and Future

Dragos Vinereanu
*University of Medicine and Pharmacy Carol Davila, Cardiology, University Hospital of
Bucharest, Splaiul Independentei 169, Bucharest, 05098, Romania*

Abstract. Atherosclerotic disease is considered to be the leading cause of death and loss of
disability-adjusted life-years worldwide. Major differences are between different countries,
mainly because of the variation of risk factors for atherosclerosis between populations.
Over 300 risk factors have been associated with atherosclerosis and its major complications,
coronary heart disease and stroke. However, between 70% and 90% of the risk of
atherosclerotic disease can be explained by different associations between conventional risk
factors, such as smoking, abnormal lipids, hypertension, diabetes, obesity, psychosocial
factors, unhealthy diet, and lack of physical activity. Because risk factors can have
multiplicative effects, their assessment in an individual subject needs application of
different models for total risk estimation. Effective cardiovascular prevention needs a
global strategy, based on knowledge of the importance of different risk factors,
conventional and newly-described, and of the best model that can be applied to assess risk
for atherosclerotic disease in an individual subject.

Keywords. Risk factors, atherosclerosis, coronary heart disease, myocardial infarction

Epidemiology

Cardiovascular diseases are the major cause of death in adults in the world, accounting for about
50% of all death and for 30% of all death before the age of 65 years. One in 8 men and one in 17
women die from cardiovascular disease before the age of 65 years [1].

There are still major differences in cardiovascular mortality between different European
countries, with high mortality rates in Central and Eastern Europe (ranging from 5 per 1000
inhabitants in Poland to 9 per 1000 inhabitants in Ukraine and Bulgaria), and relatively low
mortality rates in Northern, Western and Southern Europe (ranging from 2 to 4 per 1000
inhabitants). Trends of age and gender standardised cardiovascular mortality during the 1980-
2002 period show a similar pattern to all-cause mortality: up sloping curves in Central and
Eastern Europe (e.g. Ukraine, Bulgaria, and Romania), and down sloping curves in the Northern,
Western and Southern Europe (except Greece) (Figure 1) [2].

It should be noted, however, that while standardised mortality rates continue to decline,
the crude, non-standardised mortality rates remain stable or even increase (e.g. Ukraine, Bulgaria,
and Romania), due to the ageing of the population.

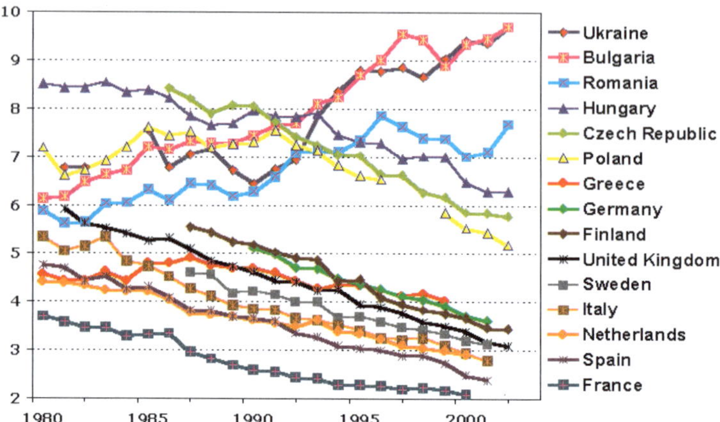

Figure 1. Age and gender standardised cardiovascular mortality per 1000 inhabitants [2] (copyright ESC: reproduced with permission).

Of the cardiovascular deaths, more than 70% are due to the complications of atherosclerosis (nearly 50% results from coronary artery disease and another 20% from stroke). Coronary heart disease is now the leading cause of death worldwide, 3.8 million men and 3.4 million women dying each year from this disease (Figure 2 and 3). Stroke is the third leading cause of death and the principal cause of long-term disability. Moreover, coronary heart disease and stroke account for 11.8% and 10.5% of all disability-adjusted life-years (DALY's) lost in men and women, respectively [3].

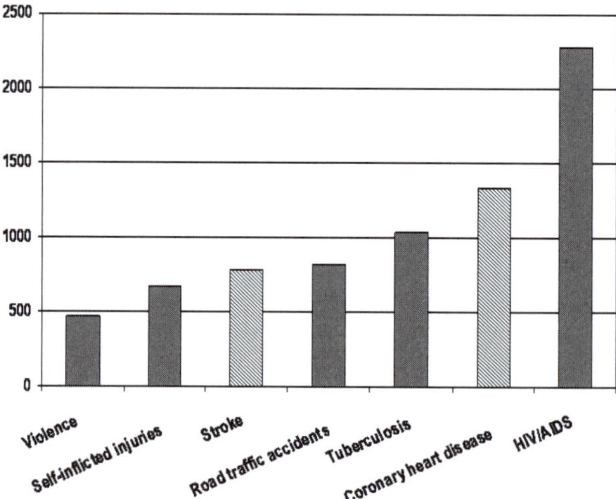

Figure 2. Number of deaths (thousands) worldwide of people aged 15 to 59 years [3].

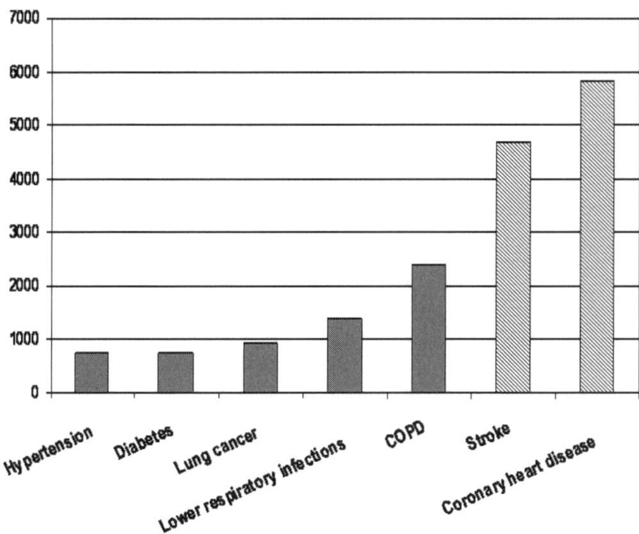

Figure 3. Number of deaths (thousands) worldwide of people aged 60 years and above [3].
COPD = chronic obstructive pulmonary disease

The main cause of mortality from coronary artery disease is represented by the acute coronary syndromes. Their clinical classification is presented in Figure 4 [4]. Of the patients enrolled into the Euro Heart Survey on Acute Coronary Syndromes, 57% presented with no ST elevation and 47% with ST elevation. Of patients with no ST elevation, 64% were discharged with a diagnosis of unstable angina, 13% with non-Q-wave myocardial infarction, and only 9% with Q-wave myocardial infarction. Of patients with ST elevation, 65% were discharged with a diagnosis of Q-wave myocardial infarction [5].

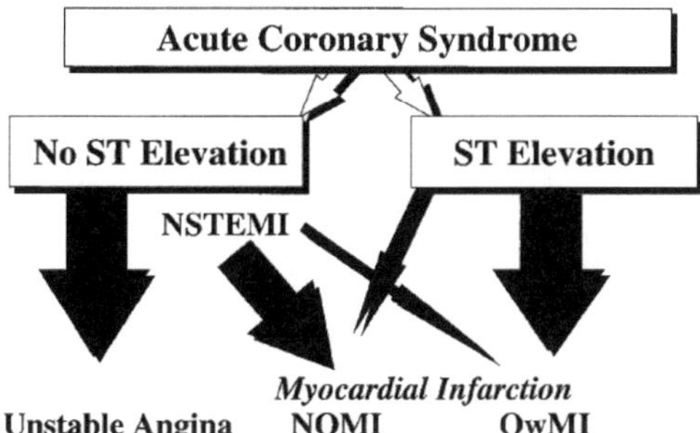

Figure 4. Clinical classification of acute coronary syndromes. NQMI = non-Q-wave myocardial infarction; NSTEMI = non-ST elevation myocardial infarction; QwMI = Q-wave myocardial infarction; ST = ST segment of ECG tracing [4].

In-hospital mortality rates were 1.0% for patients with unstable angina, 5.8% for non-Q-wave myocardial infarction, and 9.3% for Q-wave myocardial infarction. At 30 days, mortality rates were 1.7%, 7.4%, and 11.1%, respectively [6], with rather high differences between different European countries (Figure 5) [2].

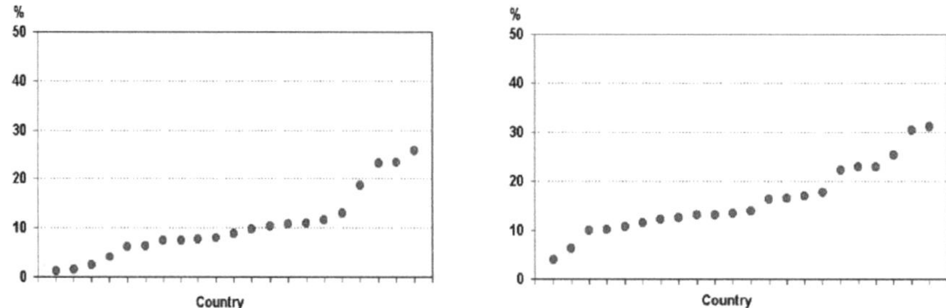

Figure 5. 30-day mortality in acute coronary syndromes admitted without *(left)* and with *(right)* ST elevation [2] (copyright ESC: reproduced with permission).

The likelihood of a person to develop a cardiovascular event due to atherosclerosis over a definite period of time (usually 10 years) defines a risk factor. There are two basic categories of risk factors for atherosclerosis: conventional, well-demonstrated, incorporated already into different risk prediction models, and newly-described risk factors (Table 1) [7]. From a historical perspective, all major risk factors were initially described by the Framingham Heart Study (Table 2) (www.framingham.com/heart/timeline.htm).

Table 1. Risk factors for atherosclerosis

Category	Risk factors
Conventional risk factors	
Predisposing factors	Age, sex, family history, genes
Risk-modifying behaviours	Smoking, nutrition, physical activity, psychosocial factors
Metabolic risk factors	Dyslipidaemia, hypertension, diabetes, obesity, metabolic syndrome
New risk factors	
Markers of inflammation	C-reactive protein and other markers
Metabolic risk factors	Homocysteine, lipoprotein(a)
Thrombogenic factors	Fibrinogen, fibrin D-dimer, markers of fibrinolytic function, other risk factors for arterial thrombosis
Markers of sub-clinical atherosclerosis	Markers of endothelial dysfunction, arterial stiffness, intima-media thickness, ankle-brachial index, calcium score

Table 2. A timeline of milestones from the Framingham Heart Study

Year	Milestone
1948	Start of the Framingham Heart Study
1960	Smoking found to increase the risk of heart disease
1961	Cholesterol level and blood pressure found to increase the risk of heart disease
1967	Physical activity found to reduce the risk of heart disease Obesity found to increase the risk of heart disease
1974	Diabetes found to increase the risk of heart disease
1978	Psychosocial factors found to increase the risk of heart diseases
1981	Major report issued on relationship of diet and heart disease
1990	Homocysteine suggested to be a possible risk factor for heart disease
1994	Lipoprotein(a) suggested to be a possible risk factor for heart disease
1998	New risk prediction model described to calculate risk of a subject for developing coronary disease

Conventional Risk Factors

1. Predisposing Factors

1.1. Age and Sex

Coronary heart disease is related strongly to age. Europe has the oldest population in the world, with a projection of one in three Europeans aged 65 and over by 2050 [1,4].

Therefore, the prevalence of patients who are at risk is on the increase and the overall burden of coronary heart disease is anticipated to increase in the forthcoming decades.

Female gender is considered as a protection against coronary heart disease. The age-specific incidence rates are 3-6 times lower in women compared to men, but this difference attenuates at older age [8]. Moreover, in younger patients with acute coronary syndromes, women were less likely than men to present with ST elevation, however, in older patients there were no differences [9]. The onset of coronary heart disease events may be delayed by some 10 years in women, but when they are affected by the disease their prognosis is worse [1].

1.2. Family History and Genetic Factors

The importance of a family history as a risk factor for coronary heart disease has been established: (1) when an individual is a first degree relative of a family member who has developed coronary heart disease; (2) when the percentage of family members with coronary heart disease is increased; (3) when family members developed coronary heart disease at young ages [1]. Lifestyle advice and, where appropriate, therapeutic management of the other risk factors should be used for members of families where coronary heart disease is highly prevalent.

A large number of genes have been investigated in relation to the risk of coronary heart disease. Apart from some well-defined genetic disorders, such as familial hypercholesterolaemia and familial combined hyperlipidaemia, which are strongly related to severe atherosclerosis and premature coronary heart disease, there is also evidence of a relatively important genetic contribution to some of the major risk factors of atherosclerosis.

This genetic contribution is usually estimated by "heritability". And indeed, for apolipoproteins and lipid traits heritability varies between 40-60% [10], and for plasma lipoprotein(a) heritability is reported to be >90% [11]. So far, however, DNA-based tests do not add significantly to the assessment of overall risk of atherosclerosis [1].

2. Risk-Modifying Behaviours

2.1. Smoking

Smoking is the most important modifiable risk factor for coronary heart disease. A strong and graded relation was found between dose (number of cigarettes smoked) and risk of myocardial infarction, with the risk increasing at every increment, so that subjects smoking more than 40 cigarettes per day had an OR of 9.16 (99% CI 6.18-13.58) (Figure 6) [12].

The risk is particularly high if smoking starts before the age of 16 years [3]. Smoking acts synergistically with the other risk factors, and also with oral contraceptive agents, placing smoking women taking this medication at even higher risk [1].

There are now nearly 1 billion individuals smoking worldwide [3]. Within Europe, the impact of smoking has been found to be smaller in Mediterranean populations than in Northern European populations [1]. Even non-smokers exposed to environmental smoke have also a relative risk of coronary heart disease of 1.25 (95% CI 1.17-1.32), as compared with non-smokers not exposed to smoke [13].

Smoking increases the risk of atherosclerosis by several mechanisms: (1) decreases myocardial oxygen supply; (2) has acute unfavourable effects on blood pressure; (3) enhances oxidation of LDL cholesterol; (4) impairs endothelial function; and (5) has adverse inflammatory and thrombotic effects [7].

Smoking cessation reduced coronary heart disease mortality by 36% as compared with mortality in subjects who continued smoking, an effect that was consistent regardless of age, sex, or country of origin [14].

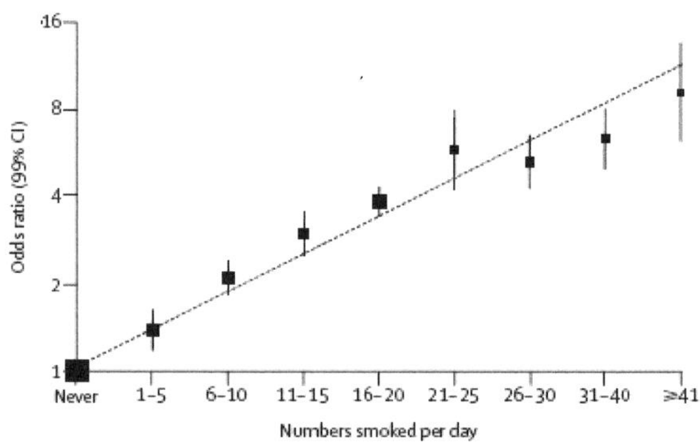

Figure 6. Odds ratio of myocardial infarction according to number of cigarettes smoked [12].

2.2. Nutrition

Nutrition, as a risk factor for atherosclerosis, includes the effects of saturated fatty acids and cholesterol, and the protective effects of polyunsaturated fatty acids (PUFAs), fruits and vegetables, and alcohol.

Food lipids are made up of 3 major classes of fatty acids: saturated, monounsaturated, and polyunsaturated, classification based on the number of double bonds between carbon atoms. In food, these fatty acids are mixed together, making the study of the effects of specific classes considerably complex.

It has been demonstrated that only the saturated fatty acids increases the concentration of LDL cholesterol and are related to coronary mortality. The source of saturated fatty acids in human diet are mainly derived from animal products, oils used for cooking or ready-cooked meals from the food industry (i.e. coconut and palm oils), and some home cooking fats (lard, hard margarines) [1]. The effect of replacing dietary saturated fats with polyunsaturated fats consists of a decrease of total cholesterol by 0.39 mmol/l and a decrease of LDL cholesterol by 0.29 mmol/l [15].

The effects of monounsaturated fatty acids on coronary heart disease are not well-established yet. On the contrary, the protective effects of some of the polyunsaturated fatty acids (PUFAs) are clearly demonstrated. And indeed, both groups of omega-3 PUFAs, of vegetable origin (α-linolenic acid) and fish oils (eicosapentaenoic acid, EPA, and docosahexaenoic acid, DHA), were shown to decrease coronary mortality and all-cause mortality. Thus, in secondary prevention, a reduction of 65% and 56% in coronary and all-causes mortality was achieved after 3.8 years, among patients randomly assigned to a Mediterranean diet, enriched in omega-3 PUFAs, compared to a control diet [16]. Moreover, in myocardial infarction, the DART study showed a reduction of 32% and 29% in coronary and all-cause mortality after 2 years follow-up, in patients eating fish twice a week [17].

Trans fatty acids are isomers, derived from meat, dairy products, margarines and ready-cooked meals, whose conformation has been modified during the digestion of ruminants or by industrial hydrogenation processes. They increase LDL cholesterol and, to a lesser extent, reduce HDL cholesterol. Epidemiological studies have found significant association between the intake of trans fatty acids and cardiovascular morbidity and mortality [1].

Fruits and vegetables are significant sources of antioxidant vitamins (vitamin E and A) and fibre. Cohort studies have shown negative correlations between the consumption of fruits and vegetables and the occurrence of coronary events or stroke. Thus, a 15% reduction in relative risk of coronary heart disease was found between the 10th and the 90th centile of fruit and vegetable consumption (indicating a 4-fold difference in fruit and a 2-fold difference in vegetable consumption) [18]. However, intervention trials of antioxidant vitamin supplements have failed to show any beneficial effects on total or coronary mortality [1,7].

Epidemiological studies showed that non-alcohol drinkers have a slightly higher risk of coronary heart disease than moderate drinkers. Indeed, in the INTERHEART study, moderate consumption of alcohol was associated with a reduced risk of myocardial infarction (OR 0.91, 99% CI 0.82-1.02) [12]. It is considered that the optimum consumption of alcohol ranges between 10 and 30 g per day (about 150 ml of wine, 250 ml of beer, or 30 to 50 ml of spirits), lower for women than for men because of enzymatic differences in the alcohol metabolism in women [19]. Alcohol has several protective effects, such as: (1) increases HDL cholesterol; (2) reduces concentrations of fibrinogen, antithrombin III, and increases concentrations of plasminogen and of the tissue factor activator, thus modifying favourably the haemostatic balance [1].

2.3. Physical Activity

Lack of physical activity is a risk factor for atherosclerotic disease whereas regular physical exercise has a protective effect. Prospective epidemiological studies have shown that a sedentary life is associated with a doubling of the risk of premature death and with an increased risk of atherosclerotic disease [1,3].

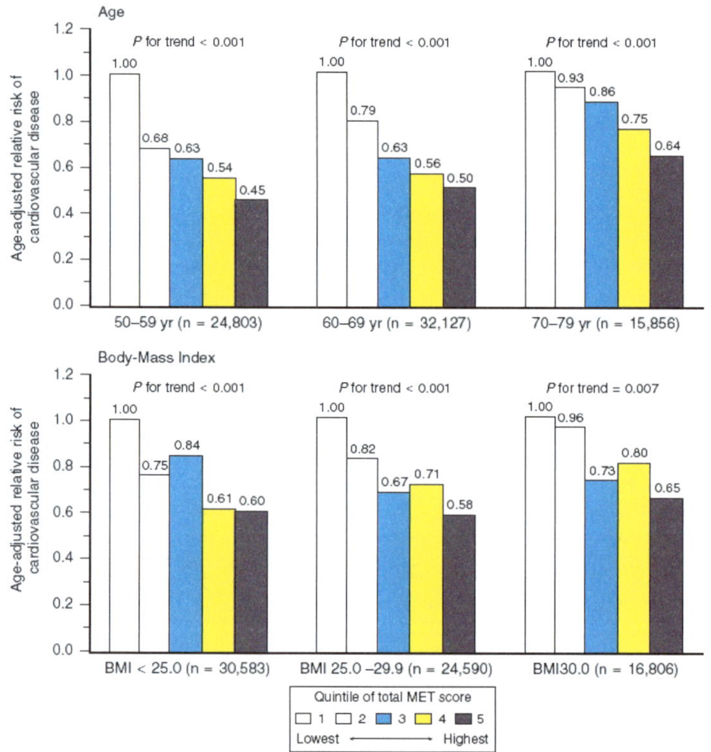

Figure 7. Age-adjusted relative risks of cardiovascular disease according to quintile of total energy expenditure due to physical exercise, measured in metabolic equivalents (MET score), in subgroups defined by age and body-mass index. The reference category is the lowest quintile of MET score (modified from [7] and [20]).

On the contrary, walking briskly for 30 minutes five times per week was associated with a 30% reduction in vascular events over a 3.5 years follow-up, irrespective of age or body-mass index, prolonged vigorous exercise being not needed for risk reduction (Figure 7) [20].

Moreover, INTERHEART study has shown that moderate physical exercise was associated with a reduced risk of myocardial infarction (OR 0.86, 99% CI 0.76-0.97) [12].

Different physical activities that have a similar benefit to atherosclerotic disease are presented in Table 3 [3]. A potential problem with a modest physical activity is that it may not be adequate to reduce weight in obese subjects. Therefore, it is now accepted that long-term weight reduction requires more vigorous exercise.

Table 3. Physical activities with similar benefits to atherosclerotic disease (modified from [3])

The following activities have similar benefits to atherosclerotic disease:
Walking 3 km in 30 minutes
Playing volleyball for 45 minutes
Bicycling 8 km in 30 minutes
Swimming for 20 minutes
Playing basketball for 15-20 minutes
Washing and waxing a car for 45-60 minutes
Washing windows or floors for 45-60 minutes

Regular physical activity has multiple protective effects: (1) it decreases LDL cholesterol and triglycerides, increasing thereby HDL cholesterol; (2) it reduces overweight; (3) it decreases blood pressure levels; (4) it improves insulin sensitivity and glycaemic control; (5) it improves endothelial function, plasma rheology, and vascular inflammation [1,7].

2.4. Psychosocial Factors

Psychosocial factors, such as low socio-economic status, social isolation, stress at work and in family life, and negative emotions including depression and hostility, have been shown to contribute independently to the risk of coronary heart disease. Thus, socio-economic status was related inversely to coronary heart disease morbidity and mortality, with a fourfold difference between the highest and lowest occupational categories. Subjects who are isolated socially are also at increased risk of dying prematurely from coronary heart disease [1]. Stress at work, such as work at night, was shown to have a 50% increased risk of coronary heart disease [21]. Clinical depression also is associated with a significantly increased relative risk of developing coronary heart disease (2.69, 95% CI 1.63-4.43) [22].

In the recent published subanalysis of the INTERHEART study, psychosocial factors were the third most important risk factor for myocardial infarction (OR 2.67, 99% CI 2.21-3.22), after smoking and hyperlipidaemia [12,23]. Subjects with high stress were younger, heavier, more often smokers, and were less likely to have a low income and a low education [23].

The mechanisms by which psychosocial factors increase the risk of coronary heart disease are complex, involving activation of the sympato-adreno-medullary system and disturbances of the hypothalamic pituitary adrenocortical axis, which affect multiple metabolic, inflammatory, and haemostatic processes [1,7,23].

Psychosocial intervention strategies and medical treatment of depression have been demonstrated to have the potential of reducing cardiac mortality and morbidity. And indeed, patients who did not receive psychosocial treatment showed greater mortality and cardiac recurrence rates during the first 2 years of follow-up, with log-adjusted odds ratios of 1.70 for mortality (95% CI 1.09-2.64) and 1.84 for recurrence (95% CI 1.12-2.99) [24].

3. Metabolic Risk Factors

3.1. Dyslipidaemia

Types of dyslipidaemia associated with atherosclerotic disease are: (1) increased LDL cholesterol; (2) decreased HDL cholesterol; and (3) increased triglycerides.

LDL transports most of the cholesterol in blood plasma, and has a strong positive association with the risk of atherosclerotic disease. LDLs are heterogeneous. Small, dense LDLs appear in plasma when triglycerides concentrations exceed 1.4 mmol/l (130 mg/dl), and they seem to be more atherogenic than larger forms of LDLs. They are associated with premature coronary artery disease, particularly in young and middle-aged people [25]. LDLs enter into the artery wall, where they are modified by oxidation, and they activate the atherosclerosis cascade. Decrease of LDL cholesterol by HMG-CoA reductase inhibitors reduces coronary events by up to 30% over a 5-year period. The goal of therapy is represented by an LDL cholesterol <2.6 mmol/l (<100 mg/dl) for high-risk patients (optional goal <70 mg/dl for very high-risk patients), and an LDL cholesterol <3.4 mmol/l (<130 mg/dl) for moderate-risk patients [26].

HDL cholesterol <1 mmol/l (<40 mg/dl) in men and <1.2 mmol/l (<46 mg/dl) in women is considered a marker of increased risk for atherosclerotic disease. HDL could ferry cholesterol from the vessel wall, augmenting peripheral catabolism of cholesterol. Moreover, HDL has also other direct protective effects, including antioxidant activity, stimulation of prostacyclin synthesis and inhibition of synthesis of platelet-activating factor in endothelial cells, and inhibition of adhesion of monocytes to endothelial cells [1,7].

Hypertriglyceridaemia >1.7 mmol/l (>150 mg/dl) is also associated with an increased risk of atherosclerotic disease, but the association is not as strong as it is for LDL cholesterol. Mechanisms involved include: (1) high triglycerides are associated with an increased level of small VLDL and IDL, which are lipoproteins rich in triglycerides, and these molecules can enter into the artery wall and follow the same cascade as LDL particles; (2) triglycerides above 1.4 mmol/l (130 mg/dl) are associated with an increase of small and dense LDL and a decrease of HDL [1]. In fact, the "lipid triad" characterised by increased concentration of VLDL and IDL, the presence of small and dense LDL, and decreased HDL has also been labelled "atherogenic dyslipidaemia" [25,26].

Since the optimal values for HDL and triglycerides are still debatable, current guidelines do not establish target values for these markers [1,26]. However, an HDL cholesterol >40 mg/dl and triglycerides <150 mg/dl are highly recommended [26].

Recently, it has been suggested that apolipoprotein B/apolipoprotein A1 ratio (ApoB/ApoA1) might be a better laboratory test for the diagnosis of dyslipidaemia associated with atherosclerotic disease, mainly because apolipoprotein concentrations are not affected by the fasting status of the subjects (unlike calculated LDL) [12]. Apolipoprotein B (ApoB) is the major protein component of LDL, IDL, and VLDL, and therefore its concentrations are a direct measure of the concentration of atherogenic lipoproteins in plasma. Values >150 mg/dl are associated with increased risk. Apolipoprotein A1 (ApoA1) is the major protein component of HDL, and therefore low concentrations of ApoA1 are, like HDL cholesterol, associated with high risk of atherosclerotic disease. And indeed, raised ApoB/ApoA1 ratio has been proved to be the strongest risk factor for myocardial infarction (OR 3.25 99% CI 2.81-3.76), with a graded linear relationship [12].

3.2. Hypertension

Hypertension is a well-demonstrated risk factor for coronary heart disease, heart failure, stroke, and renal failure. Observational studies have shown that the linear relationship between blood pressure and cardiovascular disease continues below 140/90 mmHg. Thus, the analysis of the Framingham database has proven that subjects with high-normal blood pressure (130-139 and/or 85-89 mmHg) have much higher rates of cardiovascular events than those with optimal blood pressure (<120/80 mmHg) [27].

Systolic blood pressure and pulse pressure may be of greater importance than diastolic blood pressure (Figure 8) [28]. Defined as the difference between systolic and diastolic blood pressure, pulse pressure appears to predict independently cardiovascular events, particularly heart failure. This can be explained by the fact that increased pulse pressure (probably more than 50 mmHg) is associated with stiffer arteries, and arterial stiffness is an important determinant of left ventricular function [29].

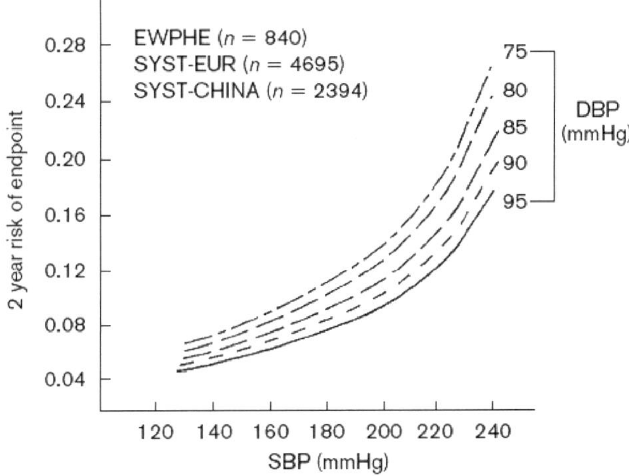

Figure 8. Risk associated with increasing systolic blood pressure at fixed values of diastolic blood pressure. The 2-year probability of a cardiovascular end-point was adjusted for active treatment, sex, age, previous cardiovascular complications and smoking by multiple Cox regression with stratification for trial (European Working Party on Hypertension in the Elderly EWPHE, Systolic Hypertension in Europe SYST-EUR, and Systolic Hypertension in China SYST-CHINA). Note that, at each given value of SBP, the 2-year risk is greater when the value of DBP is less, indicating the specific role of pulse pressure in cardiovascular risk [27].

Major trials demonstrated that a reduction of blood pressure, even a minor one (as small as 10/5 mmHg), results in clinically significant reductions in the risk for stroke (by 44%) and heart failure (by 56%) in patients with diabetes [30].

Target values are <140/90 mmHg in the general hypertensive population, with more aggressive control needed in patients with diabetes (<130/80 mm) and in patients with significant albuminuria >1 g/24 h (<125/75 mmHg). Blood pressure can be reduced by lifestyle interventions and by different antihypertensive drugs (i.e. diuretics, beta-blockers, calcium-antagonists, ACE-inhibitors, and angiotensin II antagonists) [1]. Compliance to lifestyle has been shown to be modest, particularly with regard to weight loss, and therefore more than 90% of the patients will need medication, usually with a combination of 2 to 4 antihypertensive drugs [31]. Unfortunately, despite all the efforts, the control of hypertension in most European countries remains poor (Figure 9) [31].

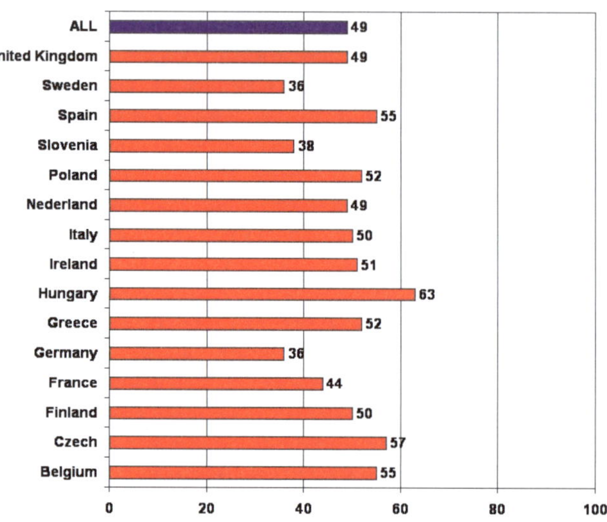

Figure 9. Therapeutic control of blood pressure (<140/90 mmHg) among those using medication (modified from [31]).

3.3. Diabetes

The status of glucose regulation is based on fasting and 2-h plasma glucose values (following a 75 g oral glucose load) into 3 categories: normal glucose tolerance (NGT), impaired fasting glycaemia (IFG), impaired glucose tolerance (IGT), and diabetes mellitus (DM) (Table 4) [32]. The major types of diabetes are type-1 and type-2. Type-1 diabetes, with the highest incidence in young adults, is characterized by loss of beta cell function with a markedly decrease of the endogenous insulin production, whereas type-2 diabetes is characterized by insulin resistance.

Table 4. Diagnostic thresholds for diabetes and lesser degrees of impaired glucose regulation (modified from [32])

Category	Fasting plasma glucose	2-h plasma glucose
Normal (NGT)	<5.6 mmol/l (<100 mg/dl)	<7.8 mmol/l (<140 mg/dl)
Impaired fasting glycaemia (IFG)	5.6-6.9 mmol/l (100-125 mg/dl)	<7.8 mmol/l (<140 mg/dl)
Impaired glucose tolerance (IGT)	≤ 6.9 mmol/l (≤125 mg/dl)	7.8-11.0 mmol/l (140-199 mg/dl)
Diabetes (DM)	>6.9 mmol/l (>125 mg/dl)	>11.0 mmol/l (>199 mg/dl)

In type-1 diabetes there is a 2-3 fold increase in the risk of atherosclerotic disease, but this is almost entirely confined to the patients developing diabetic renal disease, whereas in type-2 diabetes all patients are at increased risk [1]. Thus, the risk of developing a myocardial infarction in patients with type-2 diabetes is similar with the patients without diabetes who have already suffered their first myocardial infarction (Figure 10) [33]. Moreover, the risk of atherosclerotic disease starts to increase long before the onset of clinical diabetes. In an analysis of data from the Nurses Health Study, women who eventually developed type-2 diabetes had a threefold elevated relative risk of myocardial infarction before the diagnosis of diabetes [34].

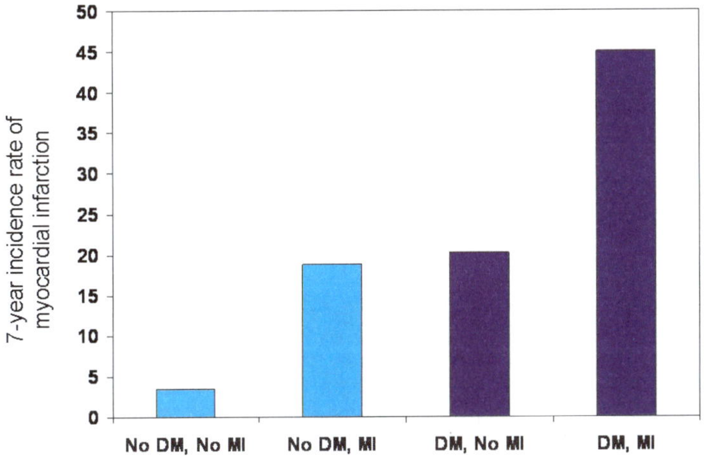

Figure 10. Risk of myocardial infarction (MI) in patients without and with diabetes (DM) (modified from [33]).

Mechanisms of atherogenesis in patients with diabetes mellitus are depicted in Figure 11. In diabetes, hyperglycaemia, excess free fatty acids, and insulin resistance increase production of reactive oxygen species, formation of advanced glycation end products (AGE), and activation of protein kinase C. These mechanisms act by diminishing the bioavailability of nitric oxide. Impaired endothelial function promotes vasoconstriction, inflammation, and thrombosis [7].

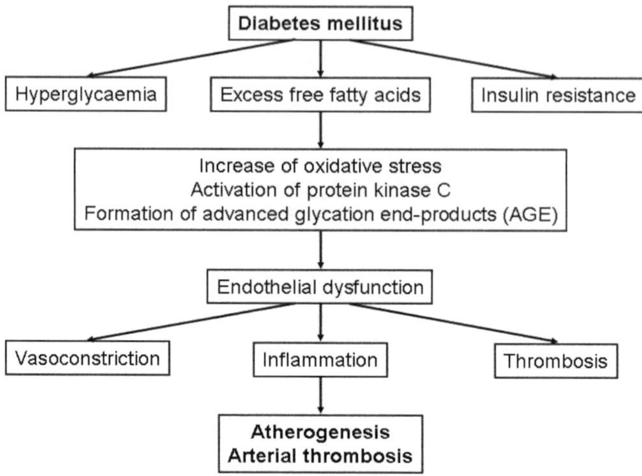

Figure 11. Mechanisms of atherogenesis in diabetes (modified from [7]).

Moreover, there is a definite relationship between diabetes, impaired endothelial and arterial function, and left ventricular dysfunction, causing the so-called "diabetic cardiomyopathy" [35]. Sub-clinical left ventricular dysfunction in asymptomatic patients with diabetes correlated with both, the glycaemic control (glycated haemoglobin HbA1c) and with lipid profile (LDL cholesterol) [36], suggesting once more that both should be targeted during management of a patient with diabetes [35].

In order to decrease the atherosclerotic risk, the treatment of a patient with diabetes should focus on the control of glycaemia, blood pressure, and dyslipidaemia. A 1% decrease of glycated haemoglobin (HbA1c) was associated with a significant 14% reduction in the risk of myocardial infarction [37]. Meanwhile, a 10/5 mmHg decrease of systolic and diastolic blood pressure was associated with a 44% reduction in the risk of stroke, and a 21% reduction in the risk of myocardial infarction [30]. Moreover, a decrease of LDL cholesterol by 40% after 2 years of treatment with atorvastatin 10 mg/day was associated with a 48% reduction of stroke, and a 36% reduction of acute coronary heart disease events [38].

3.4. Obesity

There are still controversies as to whether obesity itself is a true risk factor for atherosclerotic disease or whether its impact on risk is mediated solely through inter-relations with insulin resistance and glycaemic control, hypertension, physical inactivity, and dyslipidaemia. Some epidemiological studies have shown that abdominal obesity, measured as the waist circumference or as the waist-to-hip ratio, is a risk factor for coronary heart disease and stroke [1,7].

Abdominal obesity is more strongly associated with insulin resistance than any other adipose-tissue compartment. In addition, this adipose-tissue is metabolically active, producing different mediators of inflammation and thrombosis that might explain its risk for atherosclerotic disease [39].

3.5. Metabolic Syndrome

Although there are more than five definitions of the metabolic syndrome and, therefore, there are still important controversies regarding this entity [40], from our point of view, as a risk factor, the presence of the metabolic syndrome identifies a subject at increased risk for atherosclerotic disease and/or type-2 diabetes mellitus [39]. The most accepted criteria for the clinical diagnosis of the metabolic syndrome are presented in Table 5 [39]. Criteria for abdominal obesity have been reviewed recently [41], and lower values for people of American and European origin (≥ 94 cm in men, ≥ 80 cm in women) were suggested for the diagnosis of metabolic syndrome. Meanwhile, same authors suggested that presence of central obesity should be mandatory for the definite diagnosis of metabolic syndrome [41].

Table 5. Criteria for clinical diagnosis of metabolic syndrome (modified from [39,41])

Criterion (any 3 of 5)	Cut-points
Elevated waist circumference	≥ 102 cm in men ≥ 88 cm in women If body-mass index is >30 kg/m^2 then central obesity can be assumed, and waist circumference does not need to be measured.
Elevated triglycerides	≥ 1.7 mmol/l (≥ 150 mg/dl) or on drug treatment for elevated triglycerides
Reduced HDL cholesterol	<0.9 mmol/l (<40 mg/dl) in men <1.1 mmol/l (<50 mg/dl) in women or on drug treatment for reduced HDL cholesterol
Elevated blood pressure	≥ 130 mmHg systolic blood pressure or ≥ 85 mmHg diastolic blood pressure or on antihypertensive drug treatment in a patient with a history of hypertension
Elevated fasting glucose	≥ 5.6 mmol/l (≥ 100 mg/dl) or treatment of previously diagnosed type-2 diabetes

Regardless of the criteria used for the diagnosis of the metabolic syndrome, underlying conditions contributing to the risk for atherosclerotic disease are insulin resistance, abdominal obesity, hypertension, atherogenic dyslipidaemia (elevated triglycerides, increased small LDL particles, and a reduced level of HDL cholesterol), a prothrombotic and a proinflammatory state [39].

Patients with metabolic syndrome showed markedly increased rates of coronary heart disease, cardiovascular disease, and all-cause mortality (Figure 12) [42]. To reduce this risk, aggressive long-term management of underlying risk factors of the metabolic syndrome and of its main components is mandatory [39].

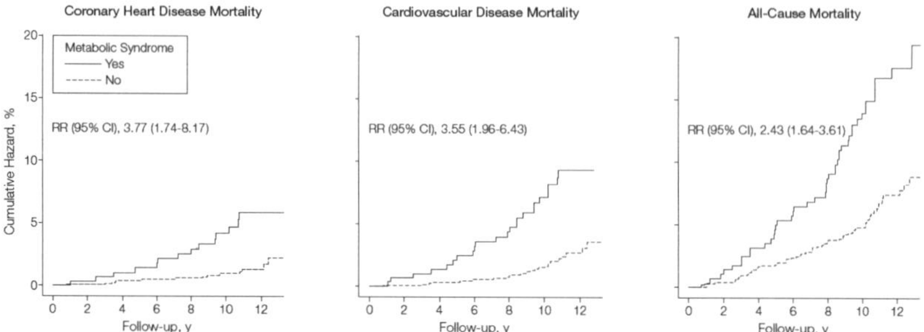

Figure 12. Cumulative hazard for coronary heart disease, cardiovascular disease, and all-cause mortality among patients with and without metabolic syndrome (modified from [42]).

New Risk Factors

1. Markers of Inflammation

1.1. C-reactive Protein

It is now well-established that atherosclerosis is an inflammatory disease. Atherogenesis involves the infiltration and retention of LDL into the arterial intima. These particles are modified through oxidation, release phospholipids, and activate the endothelial cells. Activated endothelial cells express several types of leukocyte adhesion molecules, such as vascular-cell adhesion molecule 1 (VCAM-1) and soluble intercellular adhesion molecule 1 (sICAM-1). Cells carrying counter-receptors for these adhesion molecules (i.e. monocytes and lymphocytes) adhere to these sites. Subsequent migration of inflammatory cells into the subendothelial space, through the inter-endothelial junctions, is followed by their activation. Activated immune cells migrate into the plaque and release inflammatory cytokines (interferon-γ, interleukin-1, tumor necrosis factor TNF, CD40 ligand, etc.), which induce the production of substantial amounts of interleukin-6. Interleukin-6 travels from local sites of inflammation to the liver, where it trigger the production of large amounts of acute-phase reactants, such as C-reactive protein (CRP), serum amyloid A, and fibrinogen [43].

C-reactive protein is more than a marker of inflammation. It influences directly vascular vulnerability through several mechanisms, including enhanced expression of local adhesion molecules, increased expression of endothelial PAI-1, and reduced endothelial nitric oxide [7,44].

Over-activation of the inflammatory cells can destabilize the atherosclerotic plaque. They inhibit the formation of stable fibrous caps and attack collagen in the cap, inducing rupture of the plaque, and initiating thrombus formation. Two types of proteases have been implicated, matrix metalloproteinases (MMPs) and cysteine proteases, which directly attack collagen and other components of the tissue matrix [43]. Meanwhile, massive amounts of interleukin-6 and serum amyloid A are released locally [45].

Recent studies have demonstrated that some of the inflammatory mediators can predict the risk of myocardial infarction among apparently healthy women (Figure 13) [46,47].

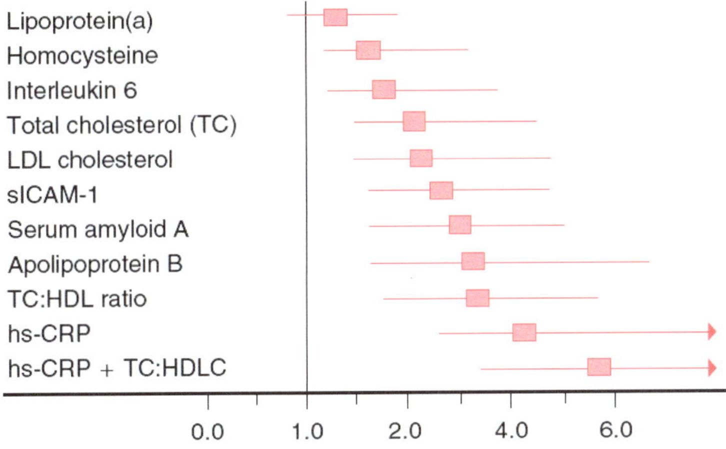

Figure 13. Relative risk of myocardial infarction for different new risk factors [46,47]. sICAM-1 = soluble intercellular adhesion molecule-1, HDLC = HDL cholesterol, hsCRP = high-sensitivity C-reactive protein.

From these markers, the best studied and the one with the highest predictive value is the C-reactive protein. And indeed, there is a large number of prospective epidemiological studies that has demonstrated that C-reactive protein, when measured with high-sensitivity assays (hsCRP), predicts strongly and independently the risk of different manifestations of atherosclerotic disease, such as myocardial infarction, stroke, peripheral arterial disease, and sudden cardiac death, among apparently healthy subjects [46]. Moreover, hsCRP adds important prognostic information in patients with other major risk factors, such as dyslipidaemia, metabolic syndrome, and hypertension (Figure 14) [48-50]. Therefore, the addition of hsCRP to these conventional risk factors provides a major opportunity to improve global risk prediction [7,51].

Based on these data, recent guidelines made the recommendation that hsCRP should be used as an independent marker of risk in patients judged by global risk assessment to be at intermediate risk for cardiovascular disease [52]. High-sensitivity C-reactive protein levels of less than 1, 1 to 3, and greater than 3 mg/l should be interpreted as low, moderate, and high risk for atherosclerotic disease, respectively. Values of hsCRP greater than 10 mg/l may represent an acute-phase response due to an underlying inflammatory disease or a recent infection, and should be repeated in 2 to 3 weeks. Consistently high values, however, should be considered as a very high risk of future acute atherosclerotic events [7,43,52]. Because hsCRP levels are stable over long periods of time, have no circadian variation, and are not affected by food intake, measurements can be done on an outpatient setting [7].

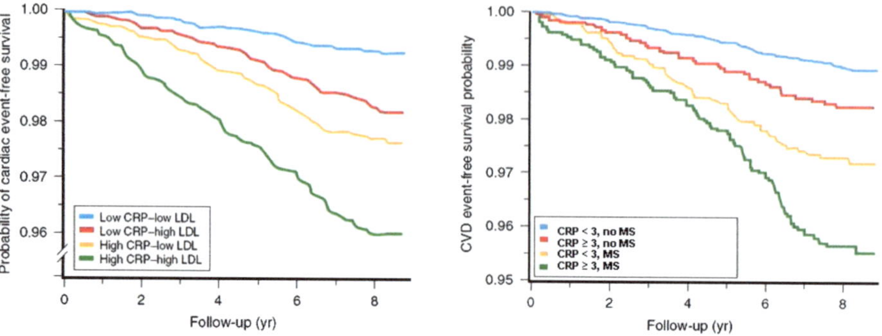

Figure 14. Cardiovascular event-free survival among apparently healthy subjects, according to levels of high-sensitivity C-reactive protein (CRP) and LDL cholesterol *(left),* and according to levels of high-sensitivity C-reactive protein (CRP) and the absence or presence of the metabolic syndrome (MS) *(right)* (modified from [7,48] and [49]).

Levels of hsCRP are decreased by different drugs, such as statins, fibrates, niacin, and thiazolidinediones [7,43]. Although it is anticipated that subjects with elevated hsCRP levels would be more likely to benefit from aggressive interventions [53], there are still no clear evidences that lowering hsCRP per se will reduce the risk of atherosclerotic disease [52]. High-sensitivity CRP levels may be useful in motivating patients to improve their lifestyle behaviours, and in taking the decision about the best treatment in some individual cases, such as prescribing statins in patients with moderate risk, LDL cholesterol below 130 mg/dl, but high levels of hsCRP [7,52,53]. However, this important question is now under direct investigation in the JUPITER study; the primary objective of this trial is to determine whether long-term treatment with a statin (rosuvastatin) will reduce the rate of first major cardiovascular events among individuals with LDL cholesterol levels <130 mg/dl (<3.36 mmol/l) who are at high vascular risk because of an enhanced inflammatory response as indicated by hsCRP levels ≥2 mg/l [54].

1.2. Other Inflammatory Markers

Other inflammatory markers have also shown promising results in terms of predicting risk of atherosclerotic disease. These include interleukin-6, soluble intercellular adhesion molecule (sICAM-1), and serum amyloid A (Figure 13) [46,47], and also P-selectin, CD40 ligand, as well as markers of leukocyte activation such as myeloperoxidase. Further research will be needed to clarify the role of these molecules as markers of risk as well as contributors to disease progression [43]. The role of fibrinogen as a potential risk factor for atherosclerotic disease will be discussed in the section 3 of this chapter.

Several studies have linked infections to chronic inflammation and the risk of atherosclerotic disease. Molecular mimicry between Chlamydia pneumoniae antigens and human molecules may contribute to the activation of inflammation. And indeed, elevated titers of antibodies against chlamydia were found in patients with coronary heart disease. However, several recent studies have failed to show that administration of antibiotics against Chlamydia pneumoniae can prevent acute coronary syndromes. Other germs under research for their possible involvement in the progression of atherosclerosis are H. pylori, herpes family viruses, and cytomegalovirus [1,43].

2. New Metabolic Risk Factors

2.1. Homocysteine

Homocysteine is an amino-acid produced by the catabolism of dietary methionine. It is metabolized rapidly during the methylation process back to methionine or catabolized to cysteine. Both metabolic pathways are catalyzed by group B vitamins, folic acid and vitamin B12 (cobalamine) in the former reaction, and vitamin B6 (pyridoxine) in the latter one [1,7]. Normal plasma levels of homocysteine are between 5 and 15 μmol/l. The measurement of homocysteine levels 2 to 6 hours after ingestion of an oral methionine load (0.1 g/kg body weight) can identify subjects with impaired homocysteine metabolism despite normal fasting levels [7]. The most frequent causes of hyperhomocysteinaemia include congenital or acquired defects of the metabolic pathways.

Severe hyperhomocysteinaemia (plasma levels >100 μmol/l) develops in patients with rare inherited defects of methionine metabolism and is associated with a markedly elevated risk of premature atherothrombosis as well as venous thromboembolism [7]. Moderate increases of homocysteine can occur as a result of a mutation in the gene coding for the enzyme methylene tetrahydrofolate reductase (MTHFR), in which cytosine is replaced by thymidine. This variant of the enzyme has a reduced activity, resulting in an elevation of serum homocysteine concentrations of about 20%. The mutation is surprisingly common, with about 10% of people in the population being homozygously affected (TT), 47% homozygously unaffected (CC), and 43% heterozygotes (CT) [55]. However, because the increase in homocysteine is relatively small and the impact of the mutation varies according to the folate intake in the population, the TT variant has only a 21% increase in the risk of coronary heart disease (OR 1.21, 95% CI 1.06-1.39) and a non-significant increase in the risk of stroke [56]. Therefore, there are no clear evidences to support the genetic evaluation of MTHFR for the prediction of risk of atherosclerotic disease [7].

Mild to moderate elevations of homocysteine (plasma levels >15 μmol/l) are detected in 5-30% of the general population, due mainly to dietary deficiencies of folic acid, vitamin B6, and vitamin B12, or excessive methionine intake [57]. Other causes include the intake of folate antagonists, such as methotrexate or carbamazepine, and impaired homocysteine metabolism due to hypothyroidism or to renal failure [7].

It has been shown that an elevated level of homocysteine is associated with an 1.3-2.8 fold increased risk of coronary artery disease or stroke (Figure 13), independent of the other risk factors, including cholesterol levels [46,56,58,59]. Meanwhile, the analysis of the Framingham study database demonstrated that plasma homocysteine levels are associated with an increased risk for congestive heart failure among patients without prior myocardial infarction (HR 1.84 in men and HR 1.93 in women) [60].

Mechanisms that can explain the negative cardiovascular effects of homocysteine include endothelial dysfunction, accelerated oxidation of LDL cholesterol, a pro-inflammatory response, and a prothrombotic effect [7,56,61].

Despite the fact that a meta-analysis reported that a 25% lower homocysteine level was associated with an 11% lower risk of coronary heart disease and a 19% lower risk of stroke [61], there are no evidences, however, that a decrease of homocysteine levels by medication, such as folic acid and/or vitamin B6 or B12 supplementation, is associated with a decrease of the cardiovascular risk [1,7]. Moreover, the recently published NORVIT study has shown that high doses of folic acid and vitamin B6 in combination may even increase the risk of myocardial infarction by 21%, despite the fact that they decrease the homocysteine level by 28% [62]. Therefore, current guidelines suggest that homocysteine measurements may prove appropriate only in a few patients, including those lacking conventional risk factors, in the setting of renal failure, or among those with premature atherosclerosis or a family history of myocardial infarction and/or stroke at a young age [1,7].

2.2. Lipoprotein(a)

Lipoprotein(a), Lp(a), is an LDL particle in which apolipoprotein B-100 is linked by a disulfide bridge to apoprotein(a), an unique glycoprotein that has chemical homology to plasminogen [63]. Although it has an uncertain physiological role, this close homology has raised the hypothesis that Lp(a) may inhibit endogenous fibrinolysis by competing with plasminogen binding on the endothelium. There are more than 25 heritable forms of lipoprotein(a), demonstrating the importance of the genome in determining plasma levels [7].

Lipoprotein(a) has modest predictive value for atherosclerotic disease by comparison with other conventional or novel risk factors (Figure 13) [46]. In a meta-analysis of 27 prospective studies, on more than 5400 patients, with a mean follow-up of 10 years, subjects with Lp(a) levels in the top third of the distribution had a risk of 1.6 times higher (95% CI 1.4-1.8) than those with Lp(a) levels in the bottom third [64]. Moreover, Lp(a) provided only a slight overall gain in prediction of coronary heart disease compared with a model using LDL cholesterol, HDL cholesterol, and triglycerides, and this gain was apparent mainly in patients already known to be at high risk (type-2 diabetes or dyslipidaemia) [7,65]. Similar results were published recently, showing that an elevated level of Lp(a) (>8.2 mg/dl) is an independent predictor of stroke and cardiovascular death in older men (65 years of age or older), but not in older women [63]. At present there is no current standardization of commercial Lp(a) assays. Finally, except for high doses of niacin, there are no other therapeutic measures that can lower Lp(a) levels [7]. Therefore, current guidelines do not recommend routine screening for Lp(a) levels [1,7].

3. Thrombogenic Factors

3.1. Fibrinogen and Fibrin D-dimer

Fibrinogen mediates the final step in clot formation, and is an important determinant of blood viscosity and platelet aggregation. In addition, fibrinogen, like C-reactive protein, is an acute-phase reactant, increasing during the inflammatory process. Therefore, it is not surprising that fibrinogen was among the first new risk factors evaluated [7].

Many epidemiological studies have reported positive associations between the risk of atherosclerotic disease and plasma fibrinogen levels. A recent meta-analysis of 31 prospective studies, including individual records on 154,211 subjects, has shown, within each age group considered, a log-linear association of the risk of coronary heart disease, stroke, and other vascular (e.g. non-coronary heart disease, non-stroke) mortality with the fibrinogen level. There was no evidence of a threshold within the range of fibrinogen level studied at any age. The age- and sex-adjusted hazard ratio per 1 g/l increase in the fibrinogen level was 2.42 (95% CI 2.24-2.60) for coronary heart disease, and 2.06 (95% CI 1.83-2.33) for stroke. These hazard ratios were reduced to about 1.80 after further adjustment for several established vascular risk factors, including C-reactive protein. The associations of the fibrinogen level with coronary heart disease or stroke did not differ substantially according to sex, smoking, blood pressure, or blood lipid levels (Figure 15) [66].

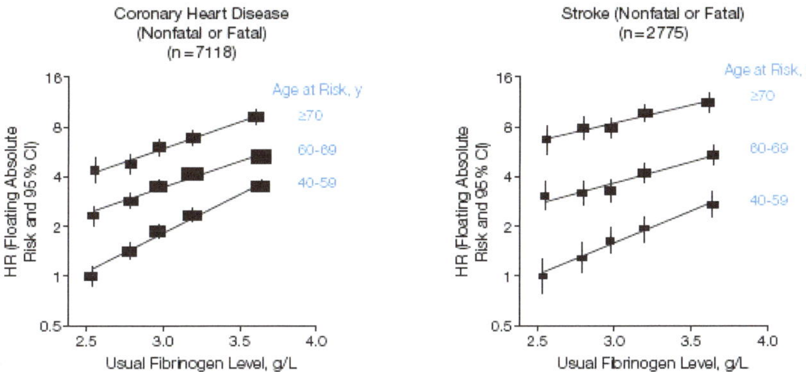

Figure 15. The age- and sex-adjusted hazard ratios for coronary heart disease and stroke by fibrinogen level [66].

Despite the consistency of these data, fibrinogen measurements have a limited use in clinical practice for several reasons: (1) the standardization of the assay is inadequate; (2) its predictive value is rather modest, by comparison to conventional risk factors and also to C-reactive protein; (3) its levels are elevated in some groups, such as women, persons taking estrogen, and smokers, thus complicating its interpretation; (4) all major studies evaluating the potential benefits of fibrinogen reduction have found disappointing results [7].

Fibrin D-dimer is the primary degradation product of cross-linked fibrin and, therefore, it can be considered as a global marker of the fibrin turnover and of the activation of the haemostatic system. In addition, in contrast to several other markers of haemostasis, fibrin D-dimer assays are more stable and more practical to measure, and therefore may be more suitable for routine clinical and epidemiological purposes [67,68]. Some epidemiological studies have shown an odds ratio for coronary heart disease between 1.7 and 2.1 comparing those subjects in the top to bottom thirds of the fibrin D-dimer distribution, but further studies are needed to determine its clinical utility [67-69]. Meanwhile, a recent study suggested that fibrin D-dimer should be examined in further research as a potential risk factor which may help to explain the differences in coronary risk between European populations [70].

3.2. Markers of Fibrinolytic Function

Endogenous fibrinolysis is regulated predominantly by tissue plasminogen activator (tPA), through the enzymatic conversion of plasminogen to plasmin. Impaired fibrinolysis, with an increased risk of arterial thrombosis, can result from an imbalance between the clot-dissolving enzyme tPA and its main endogenous inhibitor, plasminogen activator inhibitor-1 (PAI-1) [7,67].

Circulating tPA antigen and excess of PAI-1 have both been associated with atherothrombotic risk [67]. However, the clinical use of these markers for the evaluation of risk for atherosclerotic disease is low, and no data are available to suggest that the assessment of fibrinolysis adds to conventional risk scores [7].

3.3. Other Risk Factors for Arterial Thrombosis

Other risk factors for arterial thrombosis are factor V Leiden, the prothrombin gene mutation (PT G20210A), antithrombin deficiency, protein C and S deficiencies, and the von Willebrand factor.

Factor V Leiden is the most common inherited thrombophilia. It results from a single mutation in the factor V gene, causing resistance against the activated protein C, which is a physiological anticoagulant. Subjects heterozygous for this mutation have a 3 to 8 fold increased risk of venous thromboembolism, and those homozygous for this mutation have a 50 to 80-fold increased risk of venous thromboembolism. However, as shown by several meta-analyses, factor V Leiden does not appear to be a risk factor for myocardial infarction or ischaemic stroke [71-73]. Although a recent study suggested a weak but significant correlation of factor V Leiden to ischaemic stroke (OR 1.33, 95% CI 1.12-1.58), current guidelines do not recommend measurement of this factor for the assessment of risk of atherosclerotic disease [1,7].

The prothrombin gene mutation (PT G20210A) which results in increased prothrombin levels is, like factor V Leiden, associated with an increased risk of venous thromboembolism, but not of arterial thrombosis [71]. However, the same meta-analysis as above suggested that there might be a significant correlation with ischaemic stroke (OR 1.44, 95% CI 1.11-1.86) [74], but this should be confirmed by further studies.

Similarly, antithrombin deficiency is also predominantly a risk-factor for venous thromboembolism. Therefore, current guidelines recommend that evaluation for antithrombin deficiency should not be done in patients with arterial thrombosis, except in unusual circumstances [1,7].

Free protein S served as a cofactor for activated protein C in the inactivation of factor V and factor VIII. While rare cases of arterial thrombosis, particularly for protein S deficiency, have been reported, deficiencies of these proteins are predominantly risk factors for venous thromboembolism and therefore, determination of levels of these proteins should not be included in an evaluation of patients with arterial thrombosis [1,7].

The von Willebrand factor is a large glycoprotein produced by endothelial cells and also contained in platelets. It enhances haemostasis and thrombosis as an important cofactor in platelet adhesion and aggregation, and acts as the carrier protein for coagulation factor VIII. Subjects with increased levels of von Willebrand factor are at increased risk of thrombotic disorders. And indeed, a recent meta-analysis of previous relevant studies has shown that men in the top third of baseline von Willebrand factor values (>126 IU/dl) had an odds ratio for coronary heart disease of 1.83 (95% CI 1.43-2.35), compared with those in the bottom third (<90 IU/dl). Though circulating von Willebrand factor concentrations may be associated with incident coronary heart disease, further studies are needed to determine the extent to which this is causal [75].

4. Markers of Sub-clinical Atherosclerosis

Markers of sub-clinical atherosclerosis can be considered either as intermediate mechanisms between most the above mentioned conventional and new risk factors and atherosclerosis, or as direct risk factors for the complications of atherosclerotic disease. Once assessed, they can modify the evaluated risk for atherosclerotic disease of a particular subject, adding important information for its best management.

4.1. Markers of Endothelial Dysfunction

The normal endothelium, an autocrine, paracrine, and endocrine organ, plays a key role in the vessel protection against atherosclerosis, by regulating vascular tone, lipid breakdown, inflammation, vessel growth, and thrombogenesis. Conventional risk factors can promote atherosclerosis by inducing endothelial dysfunction through the decrease of bioavailability of nitric oxide (NO), which is the main mediator of the above mentioned endothelial functions [76].

A dysfunctional endothelium may lose its ability to exert its protective effect on the vascular system, and thus can be an important factor in the development and progression of the atherosclerotic process [76,77]. This is not surprising, since it is well-proven now that atherosclerosis initially involves the infiltration of LDL through the dysfunctional endothelium, followed by their oxidation in the arterial intima. The modification of LDL leads to the release of phospholipids that can potentiate the dysfunction of the endothelium, with the activation of the inflammatory process and the release of growth factors, resulting in vascular smooth muscle cell proliferation and collagen matrix production [43].

Endothelial function is most commonly measured non-invasively as the vasodilator response to shear stress in the brachial artery, a technique labelled as flow-mediated vasodilatation (FMD). Shear stress is induced by releasing a sphygmomanometric cuff after a 5-minutes over-inflation (at least 50 mmHg above systolic pressure in order to occlude the arterial inflow) at the forearm level. This induces a brief high-flow state through the brachial artery (reactive hyperaemia), which provokes the endothelium to release nitric oxide with subsequent vasodilatation, that can be imaged and quantified by high-quality ultrasounds technique. Flow-mediated vasodilatation (FMD) is typically expressed as the change in post-shear stress diameter as a percentage of the baseline diameter [76].

Although this technique assesses only the vasomotor function of the endothelium, it is attractive because it is non-invasive and allows repeated measurements [76]. Moreover, there are important data suggesting that forearm endothelial dysfunction is a marker of future cardiovascular events (Figure 16) [77]. Since flow-mediated vasodilatation is now an expanding technique, being commercially available on the new-generation echocardiographic machines, we might speculate that assessment of endothelial function will be an important step in the evaluation of the atherosclerotic risk in the near future. However, how much this technique can add to the current risk assessment scores and how it can be used to monitor treatment needs further evaluation.

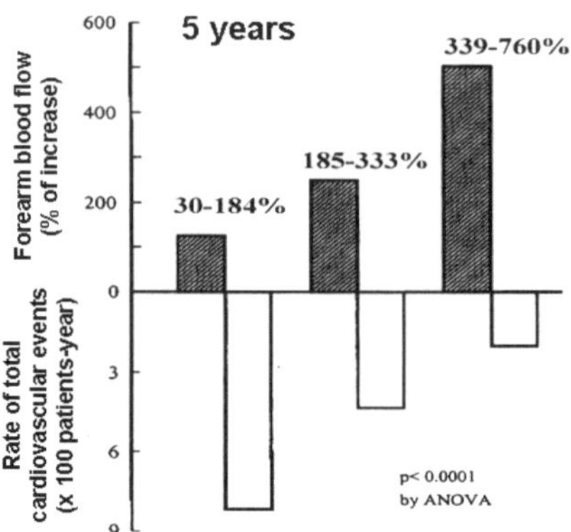

Figure 16. Rate of total (fatal and non-fatal) cardiovascular events and mean values of percent increase in forearm endothelial function, in tertiles (modified from [77]).

Another marker of endothelial function, indicating the hyper-permeability of endothelium to macromolecules, is microalbuminuria. A urinary albumin secretion of more than 10 mg/24 h (corresponding to a urinary albumine/creatinine ratio of >1 mg/mmol) is associated with a significant increase in the risk of atherosclerotic disease in the general population [1].

4.2. Arterial Stiffness

Endothelial dysfunction and incipient atherosclerosis make arteries to get stiffer and, therefore, increased arterial stiffness is now considered a marker of sub-clinical atherosclerosis.

Stiffness, or reduced compliance of large arteries, modifies arterial wave reflection timing. Ventricular ejection generates a primary (or forward) pressure wave, which moves away from the heart at a speed labelled pulse wave velocity (PWV). The incident wave is reflected from the arterial tree, generating a backward wave, travelling towards the heart. In young subjects, the pulse wave velocity is low, and so the reflected pulse wave reaches the aorta after the closure of the aortic valve. Therefore, systolic blood pressure in the aorta is unchanged, and the backward wave increases the central diastolic pressure with increase of the coronary perfusion pressure, this being the main physiological mechanism by which coronary perfusion is increased in diastole. In patients with risk factors, such as hypertension or diabetes, pulse wave velocity is increased from 5 to 20 m/s, causing an early return of the backward wave from the periphery to the aorta. This return reaches the aorta during left ventricular ejection, adding additional pressure load and increasing central systolic blood pressure, with a decrease of the central diastolic pressure and the coronary perfusion [78,79].

The consequences are represented by an increase of left ventricular afterload and ventricular oxygen consumption, associated with a reduced subendocardial coronary blood flow during diastole [80]. These mechanisms might cause left ventricular dysfunction, since we proved that increased arterial stiffness can cause dysfunction of the subendocardial muscle layers of the left ventricle [29]. Moreover, large artery stiffness has recently shown to be an independent predictor of all-cause and cardiovascular mortality in patients with hypertension [81,82]. The odds ratio of being in the group at high risk of cardiovascular mortality (>5% for 10 years) for patients with a pulse wave velocity greater than 13.5 m/s was 7.1 (95% CI 4.5-11.3) [82].

Pulse wave velocity is measured usually as the distance between two points in the line of travel of the pulse wave, divided by the time delay. Different devices are commercially available (such as Complior, Artech-Medical). Typical values range from 5 m/s to 20 cm/s [78]. Recently, new software has been available for the measurement of single-point pulse wave velocity at the level of the carotid artery. However, this software is still under validation, and more data are needed to implement it in clinical practice.

According to the current guidelines, measurement of arterial stiffness might improve assessment of the global cardiovascular risk, and might prove to be a better therapeutic target than the simple measurement of blood pressure [83]. And indeed, a recent study showed that an amlodipine-perindopril based therapy can have substantially different effects on central aortic pressure, despite a similar impact on brachial pressure, by comparison with an atenolol-thiazide based therapy. Moreover, same study suggested that central aortic pulse pressure may be a determinant of clinical outcomes and, therefore, may be a potential mechanism to explain the different clinical outcomes between the two blood pressure treatments [84].

4.3. Intima-Media Thickness

Intima-media thickness (IMT) is a marker of sub-clinical atherosclerosis at the level of the carotid arteries. It is measured by high-frequency (≥ 8 MHz) ultrasound transducers in both carotid arteries, on the distal straight 1 cm of the common carotid arteries, the carotid bifurcations, and the proximal 1 cm of the internal carotid arteries. The carotid IMT is determined as the average of 12 measurements (both sides 6 measurements each from the near and far wall of each of the three segments). A value >1.3 mm is considered abnormal [1].

Subjects without known cardiovascular disease with an increased IMT are at an increased risk for coronary artery disease and stroke. Thus, a 0.2 mm thicker carotid IMT was associated with a 33% increase in relative risk for myocardial infarction, and a 28% increase in relative risk for stroke [85]. Moreover, a recent study has shown that IMT increases with the progression of coronary artery disease, patients with mean IMT over 1.15 mm presenting a 94% likelihood of having coronary artery disease [86]. Meanwhile, in another study IMT was independently associated with the risk of stroke, with an odds ratio of 1.68 (95% CI 1.25-2.26) [87].

The measurement of IMT has the potential to improve the assessment of the global cardiovascular risk. And indeed, it has been demonstrated that the Framingham risk score increased progressively according to tertiles of IMT. Thus, with increasing IMT, the 10-year Framingham risk score increased gradually between 10% and 20% in the presence of carotid plaques, and between 5% and 20% in the absence of carotid plaques [87]. Furthermore, carotid IMT can be used as a surrogate marker in order to monitor the effects of different drugs, such as statins or calcium-antagonists, on the regression of the atherosclerotic process [85].

4.4. Ankle-Brachial Index

Ankle-brachial blood pressure index (ABI) is an easy-to-perform, inexpensive, and reproducible non-invasive test to detect sub-clinical atherosclerosis [1].

Technical requirements consist of a regular blood pressure cuff and a Doppler ultrasonic sensor. Systolic blood pressure is measured in the brachial artery in both arms, by use of the Doppler detector in the antecubital fossa. The blood pressure cuff is then applied to the ankle, and the Doppler sensor is used to determine systolic blood pressure at the left and right posterior tibial arteries and dorsalis pedis arteries. The ABI for each leg is calculated as the ratio of the higher of the two systolic pressures (posterior tibial or dorsalis pedis) in the leg, and the average of the right and left brachial artery pressures. In the case in which there is a discrepancy of more than 10 mmHg in blood pressure values between the two arms, the higher reading is used for the ABI. Pressures in each leg should also be measured and ABI calculated separately for each leg. An ABI <0.9 reflects a ≥50% stenosis between the aorta and the distal leg arteries, and progressively lower ABI values indicate more severe obstruction [88].

A recently published study has shown that, after adjustment for all conventional risk factors, a low ABI ≤0.9 was independently predictive for the risk of fatal myocardial infarction (OR 1.69, 95% CI 1.06-2.69). Moreover, the addition of the ABI increased significantly the accuracy of the predictive model for fatal myocardial infarction, by comparison with a model containing risk factors alone [89]. Therefore, ABI has the potential of being included into the cardiovascular scoring systems, with a view to improving their accuracy, but this should now be examined.

4.5. Calcium Score

Coronary calcifications occur exclusively as atherosclerotic lesions within the intima layer and are not found in healthy coronary vessel walls. The extent of coronary calcifications correlates with the extent of the total coronary plaque burden. However, the presence of coronary calcium neither necessarily reflects the severity of the coronary stenosis nor the instability of the atherosclerotic plaque [90].

Coronary calcifications can be assessed non-invasively by electron beam computed tomography (EBCT) or by multislice computed tomography (MSCT). These can be performed in a single breath hold without need for contrast medium. EBCT, however, is limited by its high cost and reduced availability, whereas MSCT has a considerably lower cost and therefore enjoys a more widespread utilization [1]. The amount of coronary artery calcification is expressed by the "Agatston score", which is a simple parameter containing the area as well as the density of calcified plaques, detecting calcium masses of ≥1 mg [91]. Other volumetric parameters, such as the total calcium volume (mm^3), the calcium mass (mg), or the calcium density (mg/mm^3) are more difficult to measure, and probably not superior to the Agatston score [1].

A meta-analysis of four studies measuring the coronary artery calcium score by electron beam computed tomography in asymptomatic subjects, and subsequent follow-up of those patients for coronary events, yielded a summary adjusted relative risk of 2.1 (95% CI 1.6-2.9) for a coronary artery calcium score of 1 to 100 (Figure 17) [92]. Moreover, a recent study has shown that coronary calcifications are a strong and independent predictor of coronary heart disease also in the elderly [93], in which they are not uncommon, being present in 29% of the men and 15% of the women without other conventional risk factors [94]. The adjusted relative risk of coronary events was 3.1 (95% CI, 1.2-7.9) for calcium scores of 101 to 400, 4.6 (95% CI, 1.8-11.8) for calcium scores of 401 to 1000, and 8.3 (95% CI, 3.3-21.1) for calcium scores >1000, compared with calcium scores of 0 to 100 [93].

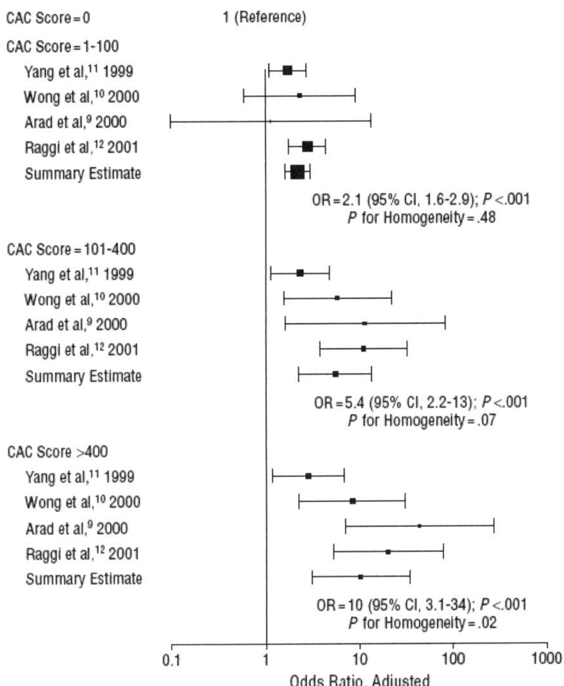

Figure 17. Adjusted odds ratios (ORs) comparing risk of a coronary heart disease event in subjects with low (1-100), medium (101-400), and high (>400) coronary artery calcium (CAC) scores to persons without calcification. Error bars indicate the 95% confidence interval (CI) [92].

Combining the assessment of coronary calcifications with the information from conventional risk factors can modify the predicted risk obtained from the Framingham risk score alone, especially among patients with an intermediate risk, which is a category in whom clinical decision making is most uncertain (Figure 18). This group of patients, with a Framingham 10-year risk score <20% and a calcium score of more than 100, might benefit from statin therapy, even at low lipid levels [90,93,95].

According to current guidelines, coronary calcium scanning should be performed in selected asymptomatic subjects, when the standard cardiac risk assessment is considered insufficient by the physician to direct further therapy plans [1,96].

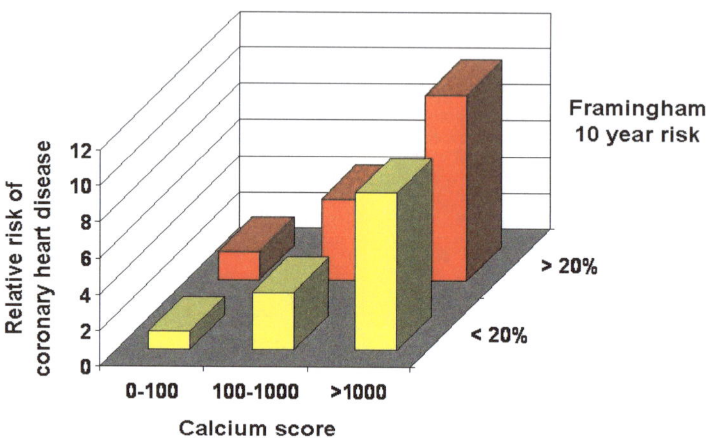

Figure 18. Relative risk of coronary heart disease by low and high Framingham risk score and calcium score categories. Compared with the reference category (subjects with a calcium score of 0 to 100 and a Framingham 10-year risk score of <20%), there was an increasing risk with increase in calcium score and Framingham risk score (modified from [93]).

Hierarchy of Risk Factors for Different Types of Atherosclerotic Diseases

The strength of risk factors for the prediction of different types of atherosclerotic diseases is different. Their hierarchy might be important, in order to apply effective prevention strategies.

The best evaluated is the relationship between various risk factors and acute myocardial infarction in the INTERHEART study [12]. INTERHEART is a large, international, case-control study, including 12,461 cases of myocardial infarction and 14,637 controls from 52 countries, representing all inhabited continents. By multivariate analysis, current smoking and a raised ApoB/ApoA1 ratio were the strongest risk factors, followed by a history of diabetes, hypertension, and psychosocial factors (Figure 19, left panel). The body-mass index was related to the risk of myocardial infarction, but this relation was weaker than that of abdominal obesity (waist/hip ratio). The daily consumption of fruits or vegetables, physical exercise, and consumption of alcohol were protective (Figure 19, right panel).

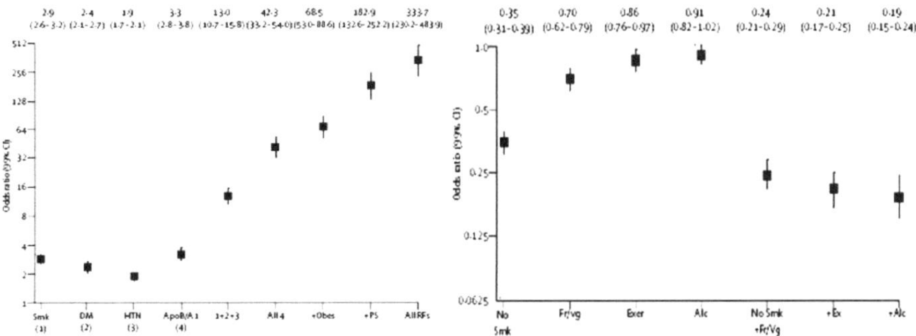

Figure 19. *Left panel:* An increased risk of acute myocardial infarction is associated with the exposure to multiple risk factors. Smk = smoking; DM = diabetes mellitus; HTN = hypertension; Obes = abdominal obesity; PS = psychosocial; RF = risk factors. The odds ratios are based on current versus never smoking, top versus lowest tertile for abdominal obesity, and top versus lowest quintile for ApoB/ApoA1. *Right panel:* A reduced risk of acute myocardial infarction is associated with various beneficial factors. No Smk = non-smoking; Fr/vg = fruits and vegetables; Exer = exercise; Alc = alcohol. Note the doubling scale on the y axis. Odds ratios are adjusted for all risk factors (modified from [12]).

Together, current smoking, hypertension, diabetes, and ApoB/ApoA1 ratio increased the odds ratio for acute myocardial infarction to 42.3 (33.2-54.0), and they accounted for 75.8% of the population attributable risk. On contrary, daily consumption of fruits or vegetables, regular physical activity, and avoided smoking conferred an odds ratio of 0.21 (0.17-0.25), suggesting that modification of these aspects of lifestyle could reduce the risk of an acute myocardial infarction by more than 75% compared with a smoker with a poor lifestyle (Figure 19) [12].

The incorporation of all nine independent risk factors, such as current smoking, diabetes, hypertension, abdominal obesity (top versus lowest tertile), psychosocial stress, irregular consumption of fruits and vegetables, no alcohol intake, avoidance of any regular exercise, and raised plasma lipids (top versus lowest quintile), indicates an odds ratio of 333.7 (99% CI 230.2-483.9). This represents a population attributable risk of 90.4%, suggesting that these risk factors account for most of the risk of acute myocardial infarction in the population [12]. The same results were reported by a systematic review on 122,458 patients with coronary heart disease enrolled in 14 international randomized clinical trials, where about 90% of the patients had at least 1 conventional risk factor [97].

Carotid atherosclerosis is responsible of more than 20% of all strokes. In the Framingham Heart Study, conventional risk factors associated with carotid atherosclerosis were age, as the most powerful, followed by smoking, hypertension, and raised blood lipids.

For peripheral arterial atherosclerotic disease (PAD), hypertension, smoking, and diabetes are the most powerful risk factors. Surprisingly, association between LDL cholesterol and PAD seems to be weaker than that for coronary heart disease; actually, the dyslipidaemia which is frequently associated with PAD is that of the metabolic syndrome and diabetes, consisting of low HDL cholesterol and high triglycerides [98].

Models to Calculate Risk of Atherosclerotic Disease in Clinical Practice

Total risk for atherosclerotic disease means the likelihood of a subject to develop a cardiovascular event over a defined period of time. Currently, there are two models to estimate the total risk, the Framingham risk model and the SCORE risk prediction model [1].

The Framingham risk model is based on the results of the Framingham Heart Study, probably the largest epidemiological prospective study in medicine. This study started in 1948 in the small town of Framingham, about 32 miles from Boston, under the direction of the National Heart, Lung and Blood Institute, and included three main cohorts. The original cohort recruited 5209 subjects, aged 30 to 62 years. In 1971, the study enrolled a second-generation group, 5124 subjects, children of the original participants. A third-generation cohort, children of the second-generation group, started to be recruited since 1990. The most important milestones of the Framingham Heart Study are presented in Table 2.

The Framingham risk model estimates the risk of an asymptomatic subject to develop coronary heart disease, defined as angina, acute coronary syndrome, or coronary death, over a 10-years period. The risk is determined based on age, sex, total or LDL cholesterol, HDL cholesterol, systolic and diastolic blood pressure, history of diabetes, and cigarette smoking. Point-based weights are assigned to the presence and/or level of each risk factor. Once the points have been assigned and summed up, their total score is translated to an estimated absolute risk of a coronary heart disease event (Figure 20 and Figure 21) [99].

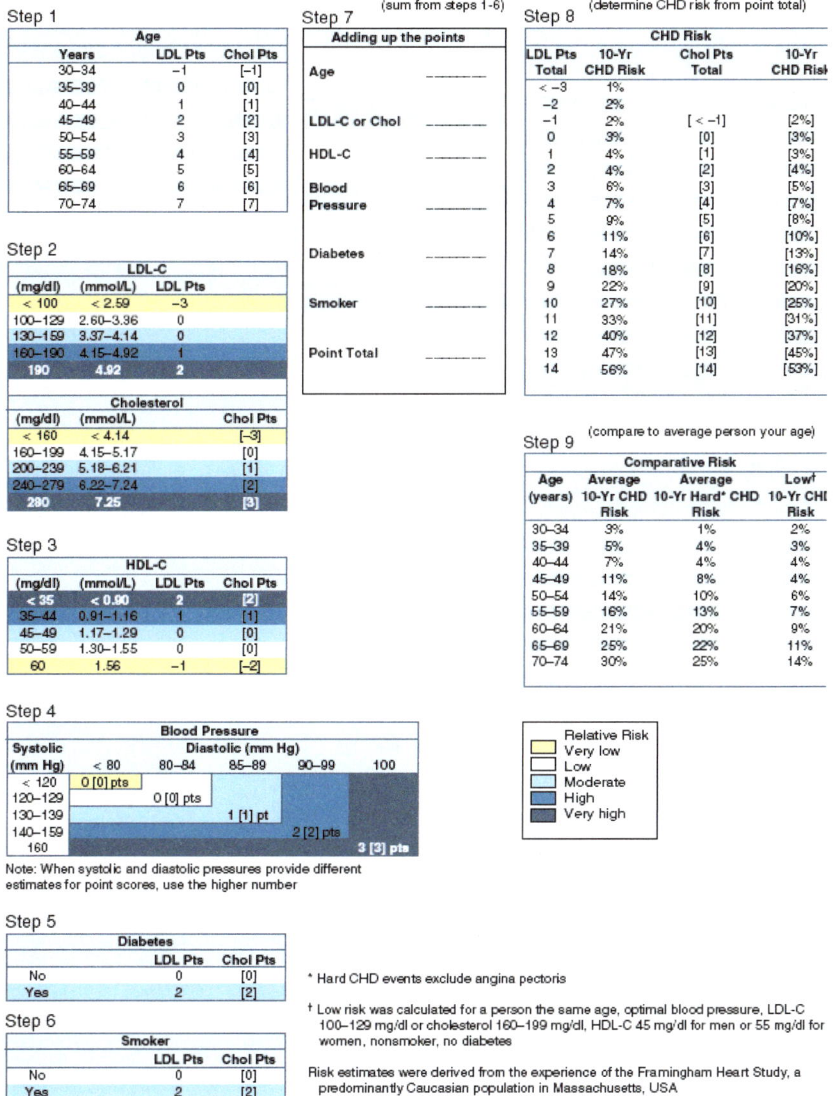

Figure 20. Coronary heart disease (CHD) score sheet *for men* using total cholesterol (Chol) or LDL cholesterol (LDLC) categories. Average risk estimates are based on typical Framingham subjects, and estimates of idealized risk are based on optimal blood pressure, total cholesterol 160 to 199 mg/dl (or LDL cholesterol 100 to 129 mg/dl), HDL cholesterol (HDLC) of 45 mg/dl in men, no diabetes, and no smoking. Use of the LDL cholesterol categories is appropriate when fasting LDL cholesterol measurements are available. Pts indicates points (modified from [7,99]).

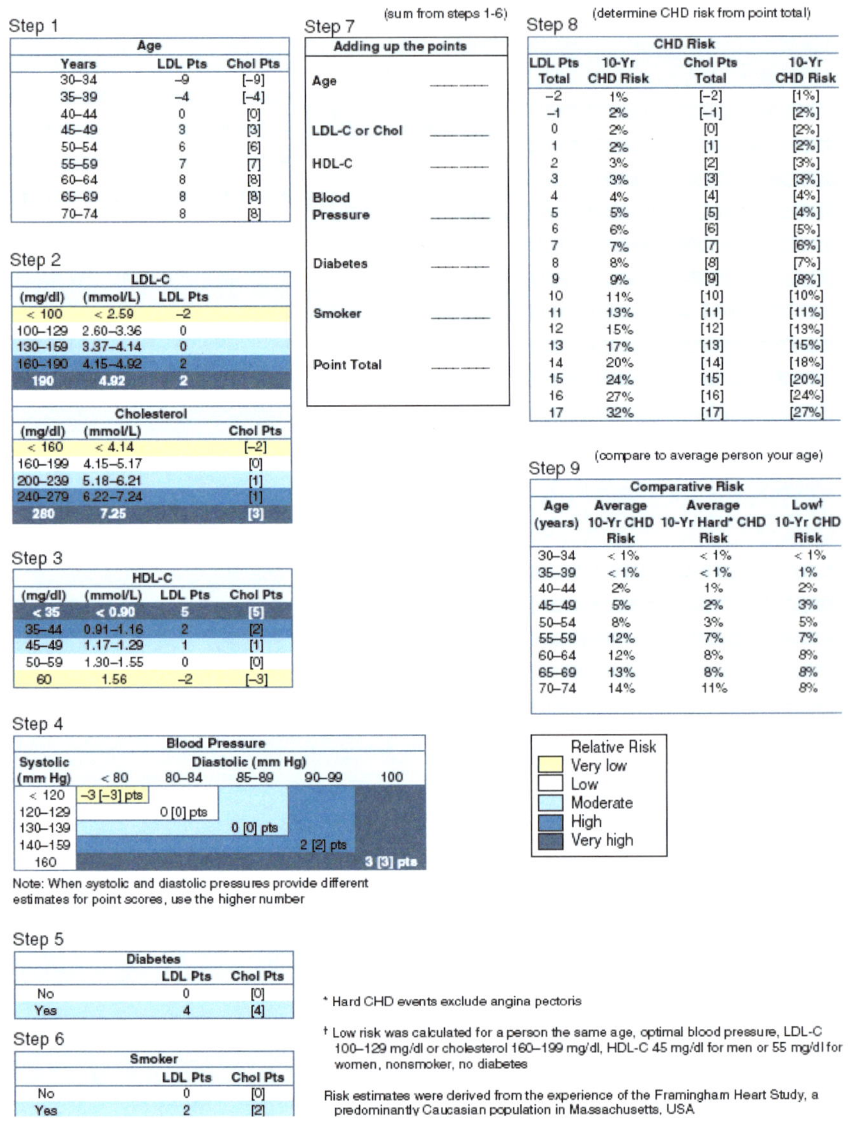

Figure 21. Coronary heart disease (CHD) score sheet *for women* using total cholesterol (Chol) or LDL cholesterol (LDLC) categories. Average risk estimates are based on typical Framingham subjects, and estimates of idealized risk are based on optimal blood pressure, total cholesterol 160 to 199 mg/dl (or LDL cholesterol 100 to 129 mg/dl), HDL cholesterol (HDLC) of 55 mg/dl in women, no diabetes, and no smoking. Use of the LDL cholesterol categories is appropriate when fasting LDL cholesterol measurements are available. Pts indicates points (modified from [7,99]).

There are several limits of the Framingham risk model: (1) it is derived from American data and the applicability of the risk chart to some European countries, such as Ireland and France, can overestimate the observed risk [100]; (2) the data set used is fairly small [101]; and (3) risk is calculated for a rather heterogeneous category, coronary heart disease, including both non-fatal and fatal end-points [101]. For these reasons, in Europe the SCORE risk prediction model was developed and implemented [1,101].

The SCORE model is derived from 12 European Cohort Studies and includes over 200,000 subjects. It has some major advantages over the Framingham risk model: (1) the primary end-point is represented by fatal events (mortality); (2) all atherosclerotic deaths (cardiac, cerebrovascular, peripheral, etc.) are included into the risk model; (3) separate charts are available for higher and lower risk countries in Europe [101].

The SCORE model estimates the risk of an asymptomatic subject to die in the next 10 years because of an atherosclerotic disease. The risk is determined based on age, sex, total cholesterol, systolic blood pressure, and smoking status (Figure 22 and Figure 23) [101].

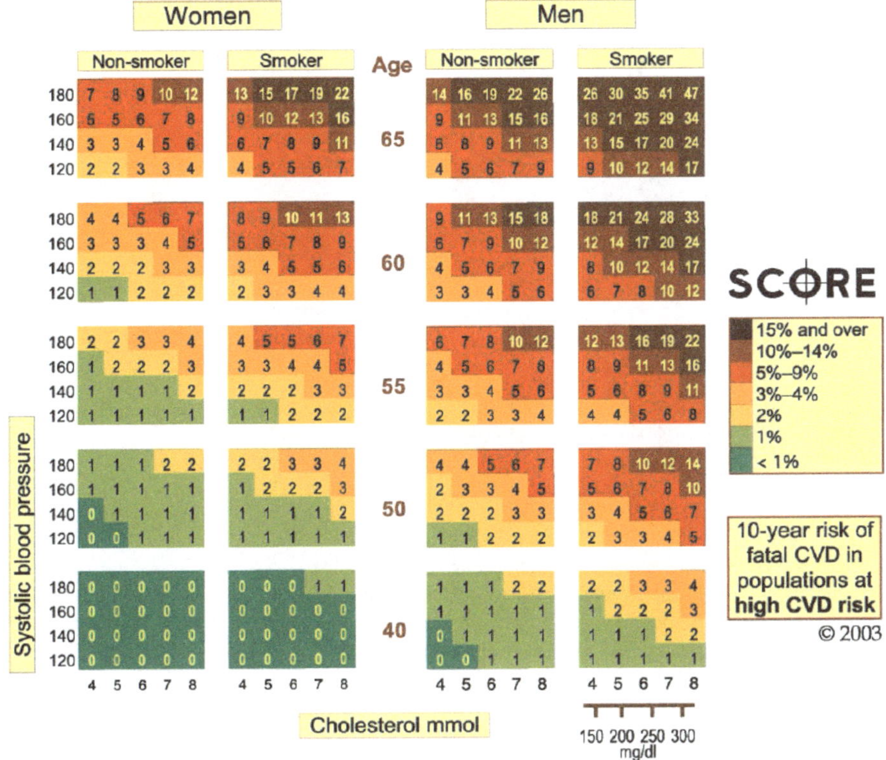

Figure 22. Ten-year risk of fatal cardiovascular disease in high-risk regions of Europe (Northern, Eastern, and Central European countries) [101].

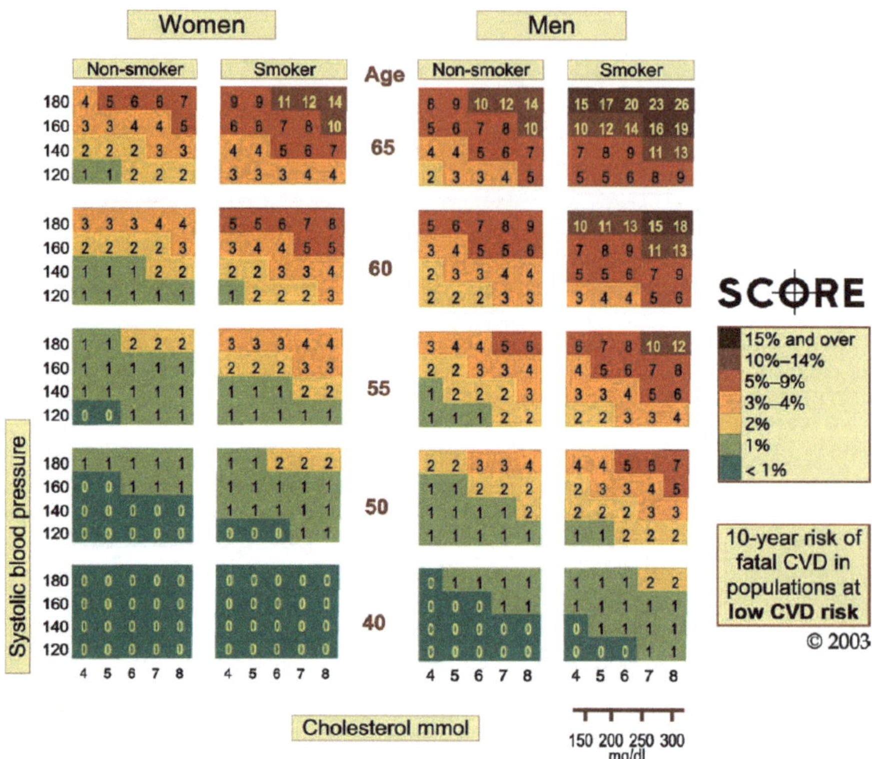

Figure 23. Ten-year risk of fatal cardiovascular disease in low risk regions of Europe (Belgium, France, Greece, Italy, Luxembourg, Spain, Switzerland, and Portugal) [101].

Conclusions

Atherosclerotic diseases, such as coronary heart disease and stroke, are the leading causes of death and loss of disability-adjusted life-years worldwide. There are still major differences in cardiovascular mortality between different European countries, with high mortality rates in Central and Eastern and relatively low mortality rates in Northern, Western and Southern Europe. Between 70% and 90% of the risk of atherosclerotic disease can be explained by different associations between conventional risk factors, such as smoking, abnormal lipids, hypertension, diabetes, obesity, psychosocial factors, unhealthy diet, and lack of physical activity. From the novel atherosclerotic risk factors, markers of inflammation are the best described, and should be probably incorporated into the further models imagined for the estimation of total risk. Similarly, new methods for the diagnosis of sub-clinical atherosclerosis should be used for the early diagnosis and for optimizing the treatment of the patients.

References

[1]　G. De Backer, E. Ambrosioni, K. Borch-Johnsen *et al.* European guidelines on cardiovascular disease prevention in clinical practice: third joint task force of European and other societies on cardiovascular disease prevention in clinical practice (constituted by representatives of eight societies and by invited experts). *Eur. J. Cardiovasc. Prev. Rehabil.* **10** (2003) S1-S78.

[2]　W.J.M. Scholte op Reimer, A.K. Gitt, E. Boersma, M.L. Simoons (Eds): Cardiovascular Diseases in Europe. Euro Heart Survey and National Registries of Cardiovascular Diseases and Patient Management – 2004. Sophia Antipolis; European Society of Cardiology (2004).

[3]　J. Mackay and G.A. Mensah (Eds): The Atlas of Heart Disease and Stroke. Published by the World Health Organization in collaboration with the Centers for Disease Control and Prevention (2004).

[4]　The Joint European Society of Cardiology/American College of Cardiology Committee. Myocardial infarction redefined - A consensus document of The Joint European Society of Cardiology/American College of Cardiology Committee for the redefinition of myocardial infarction. *Eur. Heart J.* **21** (2000) 1502-1513.

[5]　A. Rosengren, L. Wallentin, M. Simoons *et al.* Cardiovascular risk factors and clinical presentation in acute coronary syndromes. *Heart* **91** (2005) 1141-1147.

[6]　D. Hasdai, S. Behar, L. Wallentin *et al.* A prospective survey of the characteristics, treatments and outcomes of patients with acute coronary syndromes in Europe and the Mediterranean basin; the Euro Heart Survey of Acute Coronary Syndromes (Euro Heart Survey ACS). *Eur. Heart J.* **23** (2002) 1190-1201.

[7]　D.P. Zipes, P. Libby, R.O. Bonow, E. Braunwald (Eds.): Braunwald's Heart Disease. A Textbook of Cardiovascular Medicine. Elsevier Saunders (2005).

[8]　S. Sans, H. Kesteloot, D. Kromhout. The burden of cardiovascular diseases mortality in Europe. Task Force of the European Society of Cardiology on Cardiovascular Mortality and Morbidity Statistics in Europe. *Eur. Heart J.* **18** (1997) 1231-1248.

[9]　A. Rosengren, L. Wallentin, A.K. Gitt *et al.* Sex, age, and clinical presentation of acute coronary syndromes. *Eur. Heart J.* **25** (2004) 663-670.

[10]　M. Beekman, B.T. Heijmans, N.G. Martin *et al.* Heritabilities of apolipoprotein and lipid levels in three countries. *Twin Res.* **5** (2002) 87-97.

[11]　M.A. Austin, C. Sandholzer, J.V. Selby *et al.* Lipoprotein(a) in women twins: heritability and relationship to apolipoprotein(a) phenotypes. *Am. J. Hum. Genet.* **51** (1992) 829-840.

[12]　S. Yusuf, S. Hawken, S. Ôunpuu *et al.* Effect of potentially modifiable risk factors associated with myocardial infarction in 52 countries (the INTERHEART study): case-control study. *Lancet* **364** (2004) 937-952.

[13]　J. He, S. Vupputuri, K. Allen *et al.* Passive smoking and the risk of coronary heart disease - a meta-analysis of epidemiologic studies. *N. Engl. J. Med.* **340** (1999) 920-926.

[14]　J.A. Critchley and S. Capewell. Mortality risk reduction associated with smoking cessation in patients with coronary heart disease: a systematic review. *JAMA* **290** (2003) 86-97.

[15]　R. Clarke, C. Frost, R. Collins *et al.* Dietary lipids and blood cholesterol: quantitative meta-analysis of metabolic ward studies. *BMJ* **314** (1997) 112-117.

[16]　F.M. Sacks and M. Katan. Randomized clinical trials on the effects of dietary fat and carbohydrate on plasma lipoproteins and cardiovascular disease. *Am. J. Med.* **113 (Suppl. 9B)** (2002) 13S-24S.

[17]　M.L. Burr, A.M. Fehily, J.F. Gilbert *et al.* Effects of changes in fat, fish, and fibre intakes on death and myocardial reinfarction: diet and reinfarction trial (DART). *Lancet* **2** (1989) 757-761.

[18]　M.R. Law and J.K. Morris. By how much does fruit and vegetable consumption reduce the risk of ischaemic heart disease? *Eur. J. Clin. Nutr.* **52** (1998) 549-556.

[19]　J.T. Rehm, S.J. Bondy, C.T. Sempos *et al.* Alcohol consumption and coronary heart disease morbidity and mortality. *Am. J. Epidemiol.* **146** (1997) 495-501.

[20]　J.E. Manson, P. Greenland, A.Z. LaCroix *et al.* Walking compared with vigorous exercise for the prevention of cardiovascular events in women. *N. Engl. J. Med.* **347** (2002) 716-725.

[21]　L. Tenkanen, T. Sjoblom, R. Kalimo *et al.* Shift work, occupation and coronary heart disease over 6 years of follow-up in the Helsinki Heart Study. *Scand. J. Work Environ. Health* **23** (1997) 257-265.

[22]　R. Rugulies. Depression as a predictor for coronary heart disease. A review and meta-analysis. *Am. J. Prev. Med.* **23** (2002) 51-61.

[23]   A. Rosengren, S. Hawken, S. Ôunpuu *et al.* Association of psychosocial risk factors with risk of acute myocardial infarction in 11119 cases and 13648 controls from 52 countries (the INTERHEART study): case-control study. *Lancet* **364** (2004) 953-962.

[24]   W. Linden, C. Stossel, J. Maurice. Psychosocial interventions for patients with coronary artery disease: a meta-analysis. *Arch. Intern. Med.* **156** (1996) 745-752.

[25]   M. Rizzo and K. Berneis. Lipid triad or atherogenic lipoprotein phenotype: a role in cardiovascular prevention? *J. Atheroscler. Thromb.* **12** (2005) 237-239.

[26]   S.M. Grundy, J.I. Cleeman, C.N. Bairey Merz *et al.* Implications of recent clinical trials for the National Cholesterol Education Program Adult Treatment Panel III Guidelines. *Circulation* **110** (2004) 227-239.

[27]   R.S. Vasan, M.G. Larson, E.P. Leip *et al.* Impact of high-normal blood pressure on the risk of cardiovascular disease. *N. Engl. J. Med.* **345** (2001) 1291-1297.

[28]   M.E. Safar and G.M. London. Therapeutic studies and arterial stiffness in hypertension: recommendations of the European Society of Hypertension. *J. Hypertens.* **18** (2000) 1527-1535.

[29]   D. Vinereanu, E. Nicolaides, L. Boden *et al.* Conduit arterial stiffness is associated with impaired left ventricular subendocardial function. *Heart* **89** (2003) 449-450.

[30]   UK Prospective Diabetes Study Group. Tight blood pressure control and risk of macrovascular and microvascular complications in type 2 diabetes: UKPDS 38. *BMJ* **317** (1998) 703-713.

[31]   EUROASPIRE II Study Group. Lifestyle and risk factor management and use of drug therapies in coronary patients from 15 countries; principal results from EUROASPIRE II Euro Heart Survey Programme. *Eur. Heart J.* **22** (2001) 554-572.

[32]   S. Genuth, K.G. Alberti, P. Bennett *et al.* Follow-up report on the diagnosis of diabetes mellitus. *Diabetes Care* **26** (2003) 3160-3167.

[33]   S.M. Haffner, S. Lehto, T. Ronnemaa *et al.* Mortality from coronary heart disease in subjects with type 2 diabetes and in nondiabetic subjects with and without prior myocardial infarction. *N. Engl. J. Med.* **339** (1998) 229-234.

[34]   F.B. Hu, M.J. Stampfer, S.M. Haffner *et al.* Elevated risk of cardiovascular disease prior to clinical diagnosis of type 2 diabetes. *Diabetes Care* **25** (2002) 1129-1134.

[35]   D.S. Bell. Heart Failure: the frequent, forgotten, and often fatal complication of diabetes. *Diabetes Care* **26** (2003) 2433-2441.

[36]   D. Vinereanu, E. Nicolaides, A.C. Tweddel *et al.* Subclinical left ventricular dysfunction in asymptomatic patients with Type II diabetes mellitus, related to serum lipids and glycated haemoglobin. *Clin. Sci. (Lond.)* **105** (2003) 591-599.

[37]   I.M. Stratton, A.I. Adler, H.A. Neil *et al.* Association of glycaemia with macrovascular and microvascular complications of type 2 diabetes (UKPDS 35): prospective observational study. *BMJ* **321** (2000) 405-412.

[38]   H.M. Colhoun, D.J. Betteridge, P.N. Durrington *et al.* Primary prevention of cardiovascular disease with atorvastatin in type 2 diabetes in the Collaborative Atorvastatin Diabetes Study (CARDS): multicentre randomised placebo-controlled trial. *Lancet* **364** (2004) 685-696.

[39]   S.M. Grundy, J.I. Cleeman, S.R. Daniels *et al.* Diagnosis and management of the metabolic syndrome: an American Heart Association/National Heart, Lung, and Blood Institute Scientific Statement. *Circulation* **112** (2005) 2735-2752.

[40]   R. Kahn, J. Buse, E. Ferrannini *et al.* The metabolic syndrome: time for a critical appraisal: joint statement from the American Diabetes Association and the European Association for the Study of Diabetes. *Diabetes Care* **28** (2005) 2289-2304.

[41]   K.G. Alberti, P. Zimmet, J. Shaw. Metabolic syndrome – a new world-wide definition. A Consensus Statement from the International Diabetes Federation. *Diabetes Med.* **23** (2006) 469-480.

[42]   H.M. Lakka, D.E. Laaksonen, T.A. Lakka *et al.* The metabolic syndrome and total and cardiovascular disease mortality in middle-aged men. *JAMA* **288** (2002) 2709-2716.

[43]   G.K. Hansson. Inflammation, atherosclerosis, and coronary artery disease. *N. Engl. J. Med.* **352** (2005) 1685-1695.

[44]   V. Pasceri, J.T. Willerson, E.T. Yeh. Direct proinflammatory effect of C-reactive protein on human endothelial cells. *Circulation* **102** (2000) 2165-2168.

[45]   W. Maier, L.A. Altwegg, R. Corti *et al.* Inflammatory markers at the site of ruptured plaque in acute myocardial infarction: locally increased interleukin-6 and serum amyloid A but decreased C-reactive protein. *Circulation* **111** (2005) 1355-1361.

[46]   P.M. Ridker. Clinical application of C-reactive protein for cardiovascular disease detection and prevention. *Circulation* **107** (2003) 363-369.

[47]   P.M. Ridker, C.H. Hennekens, J.E. Buring *et al.* C-reactive protein and other markers of inflammation in the prediction of cardiovascular disease in women. *N. Engl. J. Med.* **342** (2000) 836-843.

[48]   P.M. Ridker, N. Rifai, L. Rose *et al.* Comparison of C-reactive protein and low-density lipoprotein cholesterol levels in the prediction of first cardiovascular events. *N. Engl. J. Med.* **347** (2002) 1557-1565.

[49]   P.M. Ridker, J.E. Buring, N.R. Cook *et al.* C-reactive protein, the metabolic syndrome, and risk of incident cardiovascular events: an 8-year follow-up of 14 719 initially healthy American women. *Circulation* **107** (2003) 391-397.

[50]   G.J. Blake, N. Rifai, J.E. Buring *et al.* Blood pressure, C-reactive protein, and risk of future cardiovascular events. *Circulation* **108** (2003) 2993-2999.

[51]   P.M. Ridker, P.W. Wilson, S.M. Grundy. Should C-reactive protein be added to metabolic syndrome and to assessment of global cardiovascular risk? *Circulation* **109** (2004) 2818-2825.

[52]   S.C. Smith Jr, J.L. Anderson, R.O. Cannon 3rd *et al.* CDC/AHA Workshop on markers of inflammation and cardiovascular disease: application to clinical and public health practice: report from the clinical practice discussion group. *Circulation* **110** (2004) e550-e553.

[53]   M.S. Sabatine and E. Braunwald. Another look at the age-old question: which came first, the elevated C-reactive protein or the atherothrombosis? *J. Am. Coll. Cardiol.* **45** (2005) 244-245.

[54]   P.M. Ridker. JUPITER Study Group. Rosuvastatin in the primary prevention of cardiovascular disease among patients with low levels of low-density lipoprotein cholesterol and elevated high-sensitivity C-reactive protein: rationale and design of the JUPITER trial. *Circulation* **108** (2003) 2292-2297.

[55]   P. Frosst, H.J. Blom, R. Milos *et al.* A candidate genetic risk factor for vascular disease: a common mutation in methylenetetrahydrofolate reductase. *Nat. Genet.* **10** (1995) 111-113.

[56]   D.S. Wald, M. Law, J.K. Morris. Homocysteine and cardiovascular disease: evidence on causality from a meta-analysis. *BMJ* **325** (2002) 1202-1206.

[57]   E.K. Hoogeveen, P.J. Kostense, C. Jakobs *et al.* Hyperhomocysteinemia increases risk of death, especially in type 2 diabetes: 5-year follow-up of the Hoorn study. *Circulation* **101** (2000) 1506-1511.

[58]   O. Nygard, J.E. Nordrehaug, H. Refsum *et al.* Plasma homocysteine levels and mortality in patients with coronary artery disease. *N. Engl. J. Med.* **337** (1997) 230-236.

[59]   D.E. Zylberstein, C. Bengtsson, C. Bjorkelund *et al.* Serum homocysteine in relation to mortality and morbidity from coronary heart disease: a 24-year follow-up of the population study of women in Gothenburg. *Circulation* **109** (2004) 601-606.

[60]   R.S. Vasan, A. Beiser, R.B. D'Agostino *et al.* Plasma homocysteine and risk for congestive heart failure in adults without prior myocardial infarction. *JAMA* **289** (2003) 1251-1257.

[61]   Homocysteine Studies Collaboration. Homocysteine and risk of ischemic heart disease and stroke: a meta-analysis. *JAMA* **288** (2002) 2015-2022.

[62]   K.H. Bonaa, I. Njolstad, P.M. Ueland *et al.* Homocysteine lowering and cardiovascular events after acute myocardial infarction. *N. Engl. J. Med.* **354** (2006) 1578-1588.

[63]   A.A. Ariyo, C. Thach, R. Tracy. Cardiovascular Health Study Investigators. Lp(a) lipoprotein, vascular disease, and mortality in the elderly. *N. Engl. J. Med.* **349** (2003) 2108-2115.

[64]   J. Danesh, R. Collins, R. Peto. Lipoprotein(a) and coronary heart disease. Meta-analysis of prospective studies. *Circulation* **102** (2000) 1082-1085.

[65]   A.R. Sharrett, C.M. Ballantyne, S.A. Coady *et al.* Coronary heart disease prediction from lipoprotein cholesterol levels, triglycerides, lipoprotein(a), apolipoproteins A-I and B, and HDL density subfractions: The Atherosclerosis Risk in Communities (ARIC) Study. *Circulation* **104** (2001) 1108-1113.

[66]   J. Danesh, S. Lewington, S.G. Thompson *et al.* Plasma fibrinogen level and the risk of major cardiovascular diseases and nonvascular mortality: an individual participant meta-analysis. *JAMA* **294** (2005) 1799-1809.

[67]   A.D. Pradhan, A.Z. LaCroix, R.D. Langer *et al.* Tissue plasminogen activator antigen and D-dimer as markers for atherothrombotic risk among healthy postmenopausal women. *Circulation* **110** (2004) 292-300.

[68]   W. Koenig, D. Rothenbacher, A. Hoffmeister *et al.* Plasma fibrin D-dimer levels and risk of stable coronary artery disease: results of a large case-control study. *Arterioscler. Thromb. Vasc. Biol.* **21** (2001) 1701-1705.

[69]   J. Danesh, P. Whincup, M. Walker *et al.* Fibrin D-dimer and coronary heart disease: prospective study and meta-analysis. *Circulation* **103** (2001) 2323-2327.

[70]   J. Yarnell, E. McCrum, A. Rumley *et al.* Association of European population levels of thrombotic and inflammatory factors with risk of coronary heart disease: the MONICA Optional Haemostasis Study. *Eur. Heart J.* **26** (2005) 332-342.

[71]   S.M. Boekholdt, N.R. Bijsterveld, A.H. Moons *et al.* Genetic variation in coagulation and fibrinolytic proteins and their relation with acute myocardial infarction: a systematic review. *Circulation* **104** (2001) 3063-3068.

[72]   K. Juul, A. Tybjaerg-Hansen, R. Steffensen *et al.* Factor V Leiden: The Copenhagen City Heart Study and 2 meta-analyses. *Blood* **100** (2002) 3-10.

[73]   R.J. Kim and R.C. Becker. Association between factor V Leiden, prothrombin G20210A, and methylenetetrahydrofolate reductase C677T mutations and events of the arterial circulatory system: a meta-analysis of published studies. *Am. Heart J.* **146** (2003) 948-957.

[74]   J.P. Casas, A.D. Hingorani, L.E. Bautista *et al.* Meta-analysis of genetic studies in ischemic stroke: thirty-two genes involving approximately 18,000 cases and 58,000 controls. *Arch. Neurol.* **61** (2004) 1652-1661.

[75]   P.H. Whincup, J. Danesh, M. Walker *et al.* von Willebrand factor and coronary heart disease: prospective study and meta-analysis. *Eur. Heart J.* **23** (2002) 1764-1770.

[76]   M.C. Corretti, T.J. Anderson, E.J. Benjamin *et al.* Guidelines for the ultrasound assessment of endothelial-dependent flow-mediated vasodilation of the brachial artery: a report of the International Brachial Artery Reactivity Task Force. *J. Am. Coll. Cardiol.* **39** (2002) 257-265.

[77]   F. Perticone, R. Ceravolo, A. Pujia *et al.* Prognostic significance of endothelial dysfunction in hypertensive patients. *Circulation* **104** (2001) 191-196.

[78]   G.M. London and A. Guerin. Influence of arterial pulse and reflective waves on systolic blood pressure and cardiac function. *J. Hypertens. Suppl.* **17** (1999) S3-S6.

[79]   M.F. O'Rourke. Wave travel and reflection in the arterial system. *J. Hypertens. Suppl.* **17** (1999) S45-S47.

[80]   S. Ohtsuka, M. Kakihana, H. Watanabe *et al.* Alterations in left ventricular wall stress and coronary circulation in patients with isolated systolic hypertension. *J. Hypertens.* **14** (1996) 1349-1355.

[81]   S. Laurent, P. Boutouyrie, R. Asmar *et al.* Aortic stiffness is an independent predictor of all-cause and cardiovascular mortality in hypertensive patients. *Hypertension* **37** (2001) 1236-1241.

[82]   J. Blacher, R. Asmar, S. Djane *et al.* Aortic pulse wave velocity as a marker of cardiovascular risk in hypertensive patients. *Hypertension* **33** (1999) 1111-1117.

[83]   M.E. Safar and G.M. London. Therapeutic studies and arterial stiffness in hypertension: recommendations of the European Society of Hypertension. *J. Hypertens.* **18** (2000) 1527-1535.

[84]   B. Williams, P.S. Lacy, S.M. Thom *et al.* Differential impact of blood pressure-lowering drugs on central aortic pressure and clinical outcomes: principal results of the Conduit Artery Function Evaluation (CAFE) study. *Circulation* **113** (2006) 1213-1225.

[85]   E. de Groot, G.K. Hovingh, A. Wiegman *et al.* Measurement of arterial wall thickness as a surrogate marker for atherosclerosis. *Circulation* **109** (2004) III33-38.

[86]   A. Kablak-Ziembicka, W. Tracz, T. Przewlocki *et al.* Association of increased carotid intima-media thickness with the extent of coronary artery disease. *Heart* **90** (2004) 1286-1290.

[87]   P.J. Touboul, J. Labreuche, E. Vicaut *et al.* GENIC Investigators. Carotid intima-media thickness, plaques, and Framingham risk score as independent determinants of stroke risk. *Stroke* **36** (2005) 1741-1745.

[88]   P. Greenland, J. Abrams, G.P. Aurigemma *et al.* Prevention Conference V: Beyond secondary prevention: identifying the high-risk patient for primary prevention: noninvasive tests of atherosclerotic burden: Writing Group III. *Circulation* **101** (2000) E16-E22.

[89]   A.J. Lee, J.F. Price, M.J. Russell *et al.* Improved prediction of fatal myocardial infarction using the ankle brachial index in addition to conventional risk factors: the Edinburgh Artery Study. *Circulation* **110** (2004) 3075-3080.

[90]   M.J. Pletcher, J.A. Tice, M. Pignone *et al.* What does my patient's coronary artery calcium score mean? Combining information from the coronary artery calcium score with information from conventional risk factors to estimate coronary heart disease risk. *BMC Med.* **2** (2004) 31-42.

[91]   A.S. Agatston, W.R. Janowitz, F.J. Hildner *et al.* Quantification of coronary artery calcium using ultrafast computed tomography. *J. Am. Coll. Cardiol.* **15** (1990) 827-832.

[92]   M.J. Pletcher, J.A. Tice, M. Pignone *et al.* Using the coronary artery calcium score to predict coronary heart disease events: a systematic review and meta-analysis. *Arch. Intern. Med.* **164** (2004) 1285-1292.

[93]   R. Vliegenthart, M. Oudkerk, A. Hofman *et al.* Coronary calcification improves cardiovascular risk prediction in the elderly. *Circulation* **112** (2005) 572-577.

[94]   H.H. Oei, R. Vliegenthart, A. Hofman. Risk factors for coronary calcification in older subjects. The Rotterdam Coronary Calcification Study. *Eur. Heart J.* **25** (2004) 48-55.

[95]   P. Greenland, L. LaBree, S.P. Azen *et al.* Coronary artery calcium score combined with Framingham score for risk prediction in asymptomatic individuals. *JAMA* **291** (2004) 210-215.

[96]   R.A. O'Rourke, B.H. Brundage, V.F. Froelicher *et al.* American College of Cardiology/American Heart Association Expert Consensus document on electron-beam computed tomography for the diagnosis and prognosis of coronary artery disease. *Circulation* **102** (2000) 126-140.

[97] U.N. Khot, M.B. Khot, C.T. Bajzer *et al.* Prevalence of conventional risk factors in patients with coronary heart disease. *JAMA* **290** (2003) 898-904.

[98] R.C. Pasternak, M.H. Criqui, E.J. Benjamin *et al.* Atherosclerotic Vascular Disease Conference: Writing Group I: epidemiology. *Circulation* **109** (2004) 2605-2612.

[99] P.W. Wilson, R.B. D'Agostino, D. Levy *et al.* Prediction of coronary heart disease using risk factor categories. *Circulation* **97** (1998) 1837-1847.

[100] J.P. Empana, P. Ducimetiere, D. Arveiler *et al.* PRIME Study Group. Are the Framingham and PROCAM coronary heart disease risk functions applicable to different European populations? The PRIME Study. *Eur. Heart J.* **24** (2003) 1903-1911.

[101] R.M. Conroy, K. Pyorala, A.P. Fitzgerald *et al.* SCORE project group. Estimation of ten-year risk of fatal cardiovascular disease in Europe: the SCORE project. *Eur. Heart J.* **24** (2003) 987-1003.

Microdetermination of Fatty Acids by Gas Chromatography
and
Cardiovascular Risk Stratification by the "EPA+DHA Level"

Heinz Rupp, Thomas P. Rupp, Daniela Wagner, Peter Alter & Bernhard Maisch
*Molecular Cardiology Laboratory, Department of Internal Medicine and Cardiology,
Philipps University of Marburg, Karl-von-Frisch-Strasse 1, D-35033 Marburg, Germany*

Abstract. The therapeutic options for interfering with the electrical instability of a pathologically remodeled or ischaemic heart remain limited. Of increasing importance become interventions which target the fatty acid composition of blood and membrane lipids. In particular, the long-chain omega-3 fatty acids eicosapentaenoic acid (EPA) and docosahexaenoic acid (DHA) provide parameters for stratification of risks associated with severe arrhythmia disorders and sudden cardiac death. Since EPA and DHA appear to have their anti-arrhythmogenic actions when present as free fatty acids, the parameters which determine a critical free fatty acid concentration are of great interest. In the present study, conclusions on EPA and DHA incorporation in blood lipids are derived from the administration of OMACOR[®] which contains highly purified (84%) EPA and DHA ethyl esters and reduced the risk of sudden cardiac death by 45% in post-myocardial infarction patients (GISSI-Prevention study). The "EPA+DHA level" is described as risk identifying parameter for severe arrhythmia disorders, particularly if they are associated with myocardial ischaemia. It appears essential not only to build up body stores for release of EPA and DHA but to provide also a sustained uptake of EPA and DHA in the form of ethyl esters. In contrast to more rapidly absorbed triacylglycerols from fish, ethyl esters are taken up slowly within 24 h. For the administration of 1 g/day OMACOR[®] to healthy volunteers, it is shown that in whole blood EPA is increased from 0.6% to 1.4% within 10 days while DHA is increased from 2.9% to 4.3%. After withdrawal, the EPA and DHA levels approach baseline values within 10 days. A gas chromatographic procedure was established which requires only 10 µl of whole blood for the identification of more than 30 fatty acids. Evidence is summarized strengthening the concept that a low "EPA+DHA level" presents a risk for severe arrhythmia disorders and sudden cardiac death. The administration of 840 mg/day of EPA and DHA ethyl esters raises the "EPA+DHA level" to approximately 6% that is associated with protection from sudden cardiac death. The pharmacological effects of ethyl esters are compared with the naturally occurring EPA and DHA triacylglycerols present in fish or fish oils which are of interest in primary prevention of cardiovascular disorders.

Keywords. Omega-3 fatty acids, EPA, DHA, OMACOR[®], sudden cardiac death, arrhythmia, fatty acids

OMACOR[®] is a registered trademark

Introduction

The stratification of risks for prevention of sudden cardiac death (SCD) remains a challenge particularly in aging populations [1]. In addition to psychological factors including depression [2,3], a number of adverse structural and molecular alterations occur in the heart which increase the electrical instability often preceding SCD. Since left ventricular hypertrophy is a major predictor of SCD [4], an important contribution arises from the high prevalence of inadequately treated hypertension leading to pressure overloaded hypertrophied hearts. Also the well-established ECG parameters increased QRS duration and QT time [4] can be consequences of cardiac hypertrophy. Furthermore, the marked myocardial fibrosis is a characteristic of hypertensive heart disease [5,6]. It promotes ischaemia and has an adverse influence on the conduction system, which often is also reflected in an asynchrony of ventricular excitation. A prolonged QT time can arise from defects in gene expression of components of cellular Ca^{2+} handling present in hypertrophied hearts involving the Ca^{2+} pump of sarcoplasmic reticulum (SERCA2a), various K^+ channels and the Na^+-Ca^{2+} exchanger. The development of drugs, which can up-regulate the expression of the SERCA2 gene and counteract the disturbed expression of associated genes has, therefore, emerged as a promising drug target [7,8] for preventing pump failure [9] and sudden death. The risk of sudden cardiac death and ventricular tachyarrhythmias is increased further during deterioration of pump function. In patients with idiopathic dilated cardiomyopathy, parameters reflecting the risk of ventricular arrhythmias have recently been described in a prospective study [10]. Reduced left ventricular ejection fraction and lack of beta-blocker use were important arrhythmia risk predictors, whereas signal-averaged ECG, baroreflex sensitivity, heart rate variability, and T-wave alternans did not seem to be helpful for arrhythmia risk stratification [10].

Dilatation of the heart occurs in about one-third of post-myocardial infarction patients [11], which is reflected in a higher incidence of severe arrhythmias [12]. While hypertensive heart disease and its adverse consequences could be prevented by a more rigorous antihypertensive treatment, dilatation in post-myocardial infarction patients can often not be prevented due to the loss of viable myocardium. Irrespective of the aetiology, the dilatation of heart chambers increases the probability of the opening of stretch activated cation channels [13,14]. This may further enhance the electric instability arising from fibrosis, which may come about from defects in Ca^{2+} handling genes and local ischaemia. Therapeutic options for preventing SCD remain, however, limited. As shown for patients with dilated cardiomyopathy [10], adequate beta-blockade should be part of the standard treatment. While implantable cardioverter defibrillators (ICDs) have proven useful, high costs are involved at least currently. The lay rescuer automated external defibrillator (AED) requires rescuers trained and equipped to recognize emergencies, activate the emergency medical services system and provide not only defibrillation but also cardiopulmonary resuscitation [15]. The impact of AED in "public access defibrillation" programs is, however, limited, since sudden cardiac arrest usually occurs at home (nearly 80% in Maastricht area) [16] and not in public places. Thus there is a clear need for developing alternative interventions, which can counteract adverse consequences of an electrical instability of the heart.

Of particular interest are in this respect factors related to the molecular constituents of lipids in the body. While the level of blood triacylglycerols and particularly LDL have been recognized as cardiovascular risk in various trials [17], the composition of blood lipids with respect to molecular components is still underrated. Blood and membrane lipids are composed of fatty acids whose nature can vary depending on a number of dietary and neuroendocrine influences. The present study provides evidence which strengthens the concept that the long-chain omega-3 fatty acids eicosapentaenoic acid (EPA) and docosahexaenoic acid (DHA), which represent a small portion of total fatty acids, provide parameters for stratification of risks associated with severe arrhythmia disorders and SCD. It is also reviewed whether free fatty acids are involved and which parameters determine a critical free fatty acid concentration required for protective effects. The conclusions on EPA and DHA incorporation in blood lipids are mainly derived from the administration of OMACOR[®], which contains highly purified (84%) EPA and DHA ethyl esters [18,19]. The latter two have been demonstrated to reduce the risk of SCD in post-myocardial infarction patients by 45% [20]. Since the incidence of the second myocardial infarction was not reduced significantly, plaque stabilization appears not to be primarily involved.

The "EPA+DHA level" is described as risk identifying parameter for severe arrhythmia disorders, particularly if they are associated with myocardial ischaemia. Since the determination of polyunsaturated fatty acids from small biological specimens (10 μl serum or whole blood) proved to be difficult to establish and to standardize, the procedures involved are described in detail. It was also found that the numerical integration of the areas of minor fatty acids required great attention and rules for the integration are given, which should permit the standardized determination also in laboratories without previous experience in lipid chemistry.

The question is also addressed, how the EPA+DHA level can be increased to a desired level in the body and whether the endogenous production from the short-chain omega-3 fatty acid alpha-linolenic acid has a role. The focus on the dosage of 1 g/day EPA and DHA ethyl esters does, however, not imply that anti-inflammatory and lipid-lowering actions, which are more pronounced with >1 g/day EPA and DHA, are not of therapeutic relevance. The pharmacological effects of ethyl esters are compared with the naturally occurring EPA and DHA triacylglycerols present in fish and fish oils which have a long-standing interest in the primary prevention of cardiovascular disorders.

Microdetermination of Fatty Acids by Gas Chromatography

Extraction of lipids. Although lipids can be extracted with a variety of organic solvents, the most commonly used procedure involves a mixture of methanol (MeOH) and chloroform (CHCl$_3$) introduced by Folch *et al* [21]. The extraction procedure for 10 samples and the transesterification step require 3.5 h and involve the following steps:

1. Prepare stock solution of 10% butylated hydroxytoluene (BHT) in MeOH, can be stored in the refrigerator.
2. Add 5 μl 10% BHT to 10 ml MeOH (final 0.005% BHT) in glass Erlenmeyer flask.
3. Prepare extraction solution according to Folch *et al* [21] by mixing 1 ml MeOH/0.005 % BHT with 2 ml CHCl$_3$ ("Folch solution").
4. Add 30x (w/v) "Folch solution" to tissue (contains 0.033 mg C17:0 internal standard) in 1.5 ml Eppendorf tube, vortex well. In the case of whole blood, use an ultrasonic bath with ice water for 5 min.
5. Extract for 45 min in ice water using a bench-top shaker and centrifuge at 4000 RPM in a table-top centrifuge for 15 min at 4°C.
6. Transfer 200 μl of supernatant to a new Eppendorf tube and mix it with 40 μl 0.9 % NaCl solution. Shake it for 5 min and centrifuge it at 4000 RPM for 15 min at 4°C.
7. Recover the bottom phase by pipetting through the upper phase preferably with gentle positive pressure (gentle bubbling) thereby avoiding that the upper phase gets into the pipette tip. Do not withdraw more than 90% of bottom phase and do not withdraw the interface. Use a reaction vial with gas-tight Teflon[®] lined screw cap.
8. Evaporate the extract using a gentle stream of N$_2$.

Transesterification of triacylglycerols with methanol. An often used method for producing methyl esters of fatty acids involves heating with a large excess of anhydrous methanol in the presence of the catalyst boron trifluoride (14% BF_3, 86% MeOH) at 60-90°C. It was, however, reported that a selective loss of polyunsaturated fatty acids and artifact peaks can occur [22,23], which was observed also in our own experiments. We used, therefore, a base-catalyzed transesterification step which requires only mild heating conditions:

1. Prepare freshly 0.2 M KOH in dry MeOH.
2. Dissolve residue (of above step 8) in 750 µl of 1:1 MeOH:toluene.
3. Add 750 µl of 0.2 M KOH in MeOH.
4. Cap the vial and heat at 35°C for 15 minutes.
5. Cool to room temperature and add 1.5 ml 4:1 hexane:$CHCl_3$, mix.
6. Neutralize by adding approximately 100 µl 1 M acetic acid and monitor the pH by putting very small drops onto pH indicator paper.
7. Add 1.5 ml of quartz distilled water and shake until upper phase becomes clear.
8. Centrifuge at 2000 RPM in a table-top centrifuge for 5 min at room temperature.
9. Add upper phase to Eppendorf tube and let the solvent evaporate in a stream of N_2 until it has nearly completely evaporated.
10. Use 1 µl for injection into the gas chromatograph.

Gas chromatography. For gas chromatography, a model 8610C gas chromatograph from SRI Instruments (Torrance, CA, USA) and a Hewlett-Packard 5890 Series II gas chromatograph from Agilent Technologies (Palo Alto, CA, USA) were used. Both were equipped with a flame-ionization detector (FID) and used hydrogen as carrier gas. For safety reasons, the hydrogen gas was produced with H2-50XR Hydrogen Generators (50 ml/min of hydrogen gas at 30 psi) (SRI Instruments) separately for each gas chromatograph. For data acquisition and integration, the Peak Simple Chromatography Data System (SRI Instruments) with Model 302 (for up to six detectors) was used.

Methyl esters of fatty acids were separated on the SP-2560 fused-silica capillary column (100m x 0.25 mm x 0.2 µm film thickness) of Supelco (Sigma-Aldrich, St. Louis, MO, USA) for which a standard with 37 fatty acid methyl esters is available (Supelco F.A.M.E. Mix C4-C24, no. 18919-1AMP). Mead's acid (C20:3n-9) was identified with the cis-5,8,11-eicosatrienoic acid methyl ester standard from Sigma (no. E6013).

Chromatographic conditions: column oven, 140°C for 5 min, increase to 240°C at a rate of 4°C/min, hold at 240°C for 20 min; injector, 260°C; detector, 260°C; carrier gas, hydrogen at 1 ml/min; split 1:10; fuel gas, hydrogen at 30 ml/min, synthetic air at 300 ml/min; total duration of run 45 min. Data acquisition was synchronized with the sample injection by using a mechanical device which couples the injection with pushing the lever back of a microswitch resulting in its closure and the start signal (Figure 1). Gas chromatograms of the fatty acid standard, and blood cells after clotting are shown in Figure 2. The areas of the fatty acid components were calculated based on the following rules (Figure 3A):

(1) Try to draw the baseline as a continuum and as straight as possible, whereby the smallest peaks/elevations are located on the baseline or touch it continuously (arrow 1).
(2) In case the baseline is not a clear horizontal line, draw the baseline to follow the smallest peaks/elevations (arrow 2).
(3) In case of overlapped peaks, draw a perpendicular dropline from the valley to the baseline (arrow 3). Do not pass the baseline through the valley points.

Following these rules, the variability between two observers became small (Figure 3B). It should be noted that the actual percentages of fatty acids are influenced by the number of fatty acids included in the analysis. These differences in fatty acid composition are shown in Table 1 for blood, serum and blood cells after clotting for the inclusion of minor fatty acids (total 34 fatty acids) or of only major fatty acids (total 9 fatty acids).

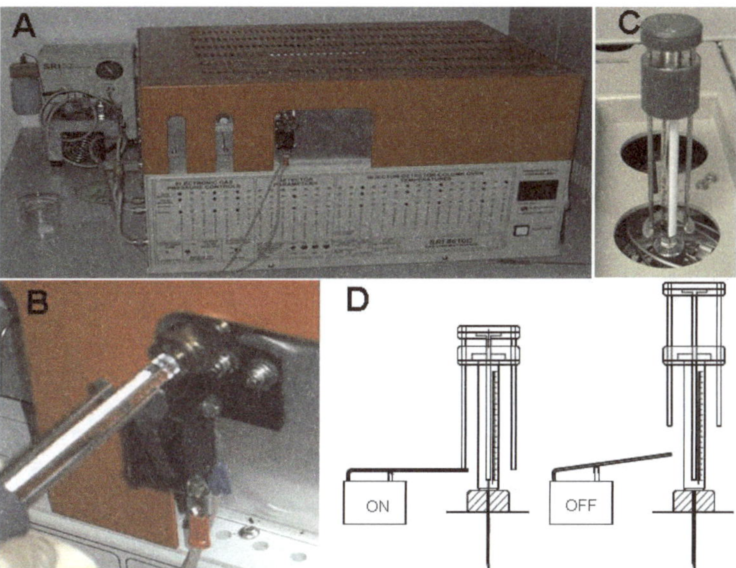

Figure 1. Gas chromatograph model 8610C from SRI Instruments (Torrance, CA, USA) equipped with a flame-ionization detector (FID). The hydrogen for the FID and for the carrier gas was produced by a H2-50XR Hydrogen Generator (50 ml/min of hydrogen gas at 30 psi) in a small quantity avoiding any risk of explosion. The model 8610C from SRI (A) and the Hewlett-Packard 5890 Series II gas chromatograph (not shown) from Agilent Technologies (Palo Alto, CA, USA) were connected to the Peak Simple chromatography data system from SRI Instruments and a personal computer. For synchronizing the data acquisition with the injection, a device (manufactured together with E. Schüler, technical development plant of Medizinische Forschungseinheiten) was used which incorporates a microswitch mounted in front of the sample injection port (B, SRI 8610C; C, Agilent 5890 II), whereby the lever of the switch was extended in a u-shaped manner (D). This u-shaped lever was pressed down during sample injection resulting in contact closure triggering the start of data acquisition. For this purpose, the syringe was incorporated in a guidance device with two thin steel rods which moved together with the needle and closed the u-shaped lever of the microswitch. This synchronization was found to be a prerequisite for reproducibly identifying fatty acid peaks based on the 37 fatty acid standard.

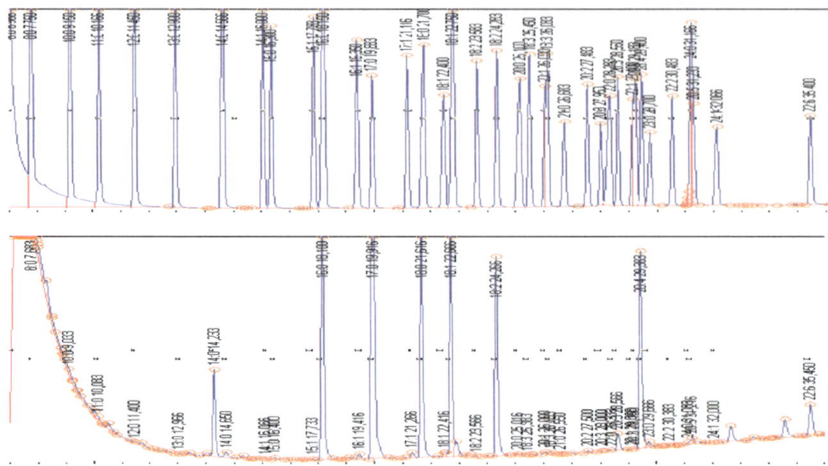

Figure 2. (Top) Gas chromatogram with 37 resolved fatty acids of a fatty acid standard (Supelco F.A.M.E. Mix C4-C24, no. 18919-1AMP). Arachidic acid (C20:0), arachidonic acid (C20:4n-6, cis-5,8,11,14), behenic acid (C22:0), butyric acid (C4:0), capric acid (C10:0), caproic acid (C6:0), caprylic acid (C8:0), cis-13,16-docosadienoic acid (C22:2), cis-4,7,10,13,16,19-docosahexaenoic acid (C22:6n-3), cis-11,14-eicosadienoic acid (C20:2n-6), cis-5,8,11,14,17-eicosapentaenoic acid (C20:5n-3), cis-8,11,14-eicosatrienoic acid (C20:3n-6), cis-11,14,17-eicosatrienoic acid (C20:3n-3), cis-11-eicosenoic acid (C20:1), elaidic acid (C18:1, trans-9), erucic acid (C22:1, cis-13), heneicosanoic acid (C21:0), heptadecanoic acid (C17:0), cis-10 heptadecenoic acid (C17:1), lauric acid (C12:0), lignoceric acid (C24:0), linoleic acid (C18:2n-6 cis-9,12), linolelaidic acid (C18:2, trans-9,12), γ-linolenic acid (C18:3n-6, cis-6,9,12), linolenic acid (C18:3n-3, cis-9,12,15), myristic acid (C14:0), myristoleic acid (C14:1, cis-9), nervonic acid (C24:1, cis-15), oleic acid (C18:1n-9, cis-9), palmitic acid (C16:0), palmitoleic acid (C16:1, cis-9), pentadecanoic acid (C15:0), cis-10 pentadecenoic acid (C15:1), stearic acid (C18:0), tricosanoic acid (C23:0), tridecanoic acid (C13:0), undecanoic acid (C11:0). (Bottom) Using this fatty acid standard, fatty acids are identified as shown for a representative fatty acid profile of blood cells after clotting.

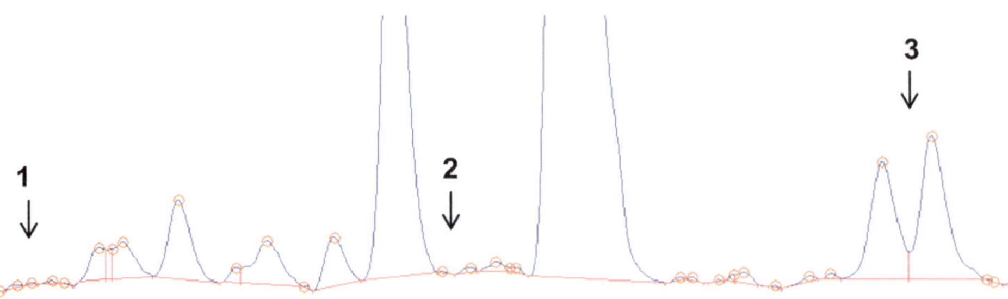

Figure 3A. Procedures for integration of fatty acids using the Peak Simple program. The arrows refer to rules described in the text.

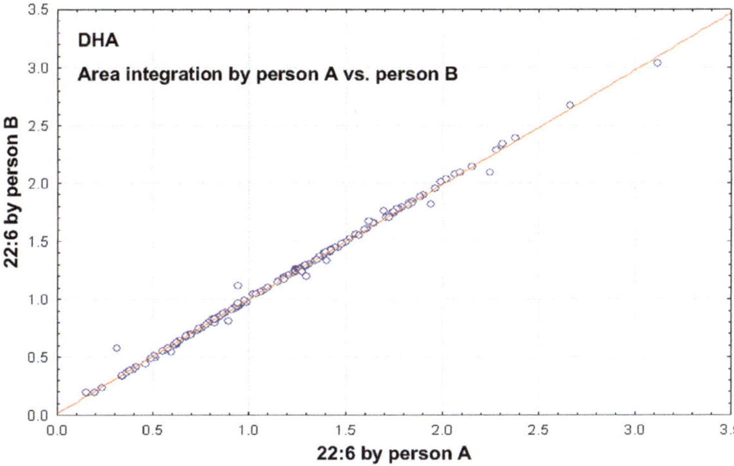

Figure 3B. Interobserver variabilities of percentage values of fatty acids determined independently by two persons.

Table 1. Differences in fatty acid composition (%) of blood arising from area calculations including also minor fatty acids (total 34 fatty acids) or only major fatty acids (total 9 fatty acids)

	Whole blood (34 fatty acids)	Whole blood (9 fatty acids)	Serum (34 fatty acids)	Serum (9 fatty acids)	Blood cells (34 fatty acids)	Blood cells (9 fatty acids)
8:0	ND		<0.05		0.1	
10:0	0.1		0.1		0.2	
11:0	0.3		ND		0.1	
12:0	0.7		0.2		0.1	
13:0	<0.05		<0.05		<0.05	
14:0	1.4		1.1		0.8	
14:1	<0.05		<0.05		<0.05	
15:0	0.3		0.2		0.3	
15:1	0.1		<0.05		<0.05	
16:0	27.9	29.8	28.0	29.4	23.7	25.0
16:1	1.0	1.1	1.3	1.3	0.7	0.7
17:1	1.0		0.1		0.1	
18:0	13.2	14.1	9.7	10.2	14.9	15.8
18:1n9t	0.1		0.1		0.3	
18:1n9c	18.4	19.7	21.4	22.4	18.5	19.6
18:2n6t	<0.05		0.1		<0.05	
18:2n6c	19.6	20.9	25.3	26.6	18.3	19.4
20:0	0.1		0.2		0.2	
18:3n6	0.1		0.2		0.2	
20:1	0.2		0.2		0.2	
18:3n3	0.3	0.3	0.3	0.3	0.2	0.2
21:0	0.2		<0.05		<0.05	
20:2	0.2		0.1		0.3	
20:3n9	<0.05		<0.05		<0.05	
22:0	0.1		0.2		0.1	
20:3n6	1.4		1.5		1.7	
22:1n9	<0.05		<0.05		0.1	
20:3n3	<0.05		<0.05		<0.05	
20:4n6	9.8	10.5	6.0	6.4	13.8	14.6
23:0	ND		ND		ND	
22:2	<0.05		0.2		0.3	
24:0	0.1		<0.05		0.2	
20:5n3	1.0	1.1	1.4	1.5	1.4	1.5
24:1	0.1		0.1		0.1	
22:6n3	2.4	2.6	1.8	1.9	3.1	3.3
EPA+DHA	3.4	3.7	3.2	3.4	4.5	4.8

Monitoring the EPA+DHA Level in Whole Blood after Intake of EPA and DHA Ethyl Esters

We conducted a study in 11 normal healthy volunteers for monitoring the EPA+DHA level in whole blood after intake of 1g/day EPA and DHA ethyl esters (OMACOR®) [24]. Whole blood had previously been used in the Physicians' Health Study examining the inter-relationship between risk of SCD and the level of omega-3 fatty acids [25]. The EPA concentration increased from 0.6% to 1.4% within 10 days leading to a plateau value (Figure 4). DHA values increased from 2.9% to 4.3%. After OMACOR® discontinuation, the values approached the pre-study level within 10 days, whereby the decline in DHA appeared to be less pronounced. The data show that within the present time scale of EPA and DHA ethyl ester administration, no EPA and DHA stores are formed in the body, which could maintain the blood EPA+DHA level after discontinuation of OMACOR® intake.

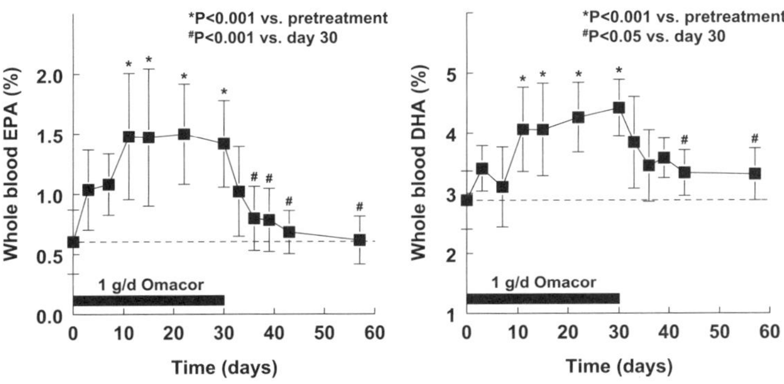

Figure 4. Whole blood levels of EPA and DHA after 1 g/day OMACOR® administration in 11 normal healthy volunteers. Fatty acids were extracted from 10 µl whole blood. OMACOR® was purchased. Statistical analysis was performed by repeated measures analysis of variance and the Tukey-Kramer multiple comparisons test using the "GraphPad InStat" package (San Diego, USA). The data are based on 11 persons during the administration of OMACOR® and 9 persons after OMACOR® withdrawal (from [24]).

The Whole Blood EPA+DHA Level and Risk of SCD

The intake of 1 g/day OMACOR® raises the whole blood EPA+DHA level from 3.5 to 5.7%. This increase is associated with protective effects, which can be inferred from previous epidemiological studies in populations with a variable EPA and DHA blood content and a link can be provided with the data of the GISSI-Prevention study [20,26,27]. While no EPA and DHA values are available for the patients of the GISSI-Prevention study, it has been reported for Italian healthy volunteers that 1 g/day OMACOR® raises EPA and DHA to levels which may explain their beneficial effects against cardiovascular diseases [28]. It is well-established that the risk of SCD is reduced when the EPA+DHA level is increased (Figure 5). In the Physicians' Health Study, base-line whole blood levels of long-chain omega-3 fatty acids were inversely associated with the risk of SCD [25]. As compared with men whose whole blood levels of long-chain omega-3 fatty acids were in the lowest quartile (2.12-4.32%), the relative risk of SCD was significantly lower among men with levels in the third quartile (5.20-6.07%; adjusted relative risk, 0.19) and the fourth quartile (6.08-10.2%; adjusted relative risk, 0.10) [25]. Also the study of Siscovick *et al* shows a risk reduction for primary cardiac arrest when the EPA+DHA level is increased [29]. Compared with a red blood cell membrane EPA+DHA level of 3.3% (the mean of the lowest quartile), a level of 5.0% (the mean of the third quartile) was associated with a 75% reduction in the risk of primary cardiac arrest [29]. Based on the data of the Physicians' Health Study [25] and the study of Siscovick *et al* [29] and our own data on the EPA+DHA level after 1 g/day OMACOR®, the reduction of sudden death risk observed in the GISSI-Prevention study [20,26,27] can be attributed to an increase in the EPA+DHA level leading to about 6% EPA+DHA (Figure 5).

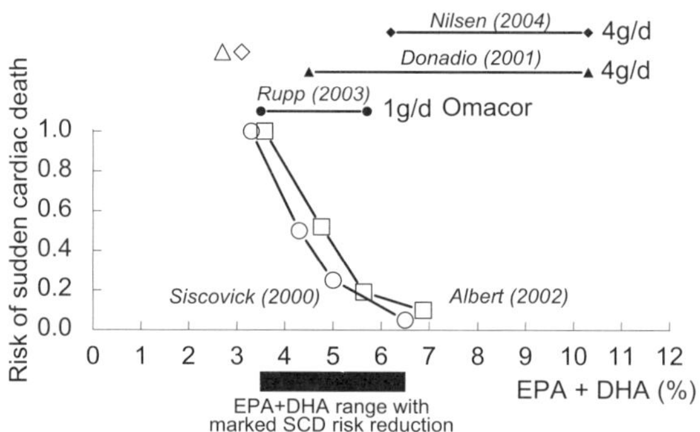

Figure 5. Inter-relationship between the EPA+DHA level and risk of SCD. Data are adapted from the epidemiological studies of (open squares) Albert *et al* [25] and (open circles) Siscovick *et al* [29]. Interventional studies with OMACOR® were performed with 1 g/d [24] and 4 g/d (Nilsen *et al* [30] and Donadio *et al* [31]). The data of Albert *et al* [25] include also docosapentaenoic acid and are, therefore, too high by approximately 0.98 percentage points. Included are also data points representing controls in the epidemiological studies of (open triangle) Guallar *et al* [32] and (open diamond) Leng *et al* [33] which are similar to the baseline values of our study carried out in Marburg. It should be noted that as in our study, whole blood was used in the study of Albert *et al* [25]. Figure from [24].

The Non-Membrane Bound EPA+DHA Level - Enhanced Release of Free Fatty Acids in Myocardial Infarction

Although it is well-known that EPA and DHA have to be present as free fatty acids before they can be converted into eicosanoids or can activate transcription factors such as PPARs [24] (Figure 6), it remains a misconception that anti-arrhythmogenic effects involve membrane bound phospholipids of EPA and DHA. Major sources for the release of EPA and DHA are phospholipid membranes (Figure 6). The polyunsaturated fatty acids EPA, DHA and arachidonic acid are incorporated to a greater extent into the inner position of membrane phospholipids [34]. A rise in sympathetic nervous system activity is associated with a raised phospholipase A2 activity and the subsequent release of fatty acids from membranes. Since phospholipase A2 mobilizes fatty acids from the inner position of phospholipids, an over-proportional increase of these polyunsaturated fatty acids is expected. This has been shown for pigs after coronary occlusion, which had been fed a diet enriched in EPA and DHA triacylglycerols [35]. Compared with pigs fed saturated fat, an over-proportional increase of the EPA and DHA concentration was observed in the raised myocardial free fatty acids. The relevance of non-membrane bound EPA and DHA is demonstrated also in a study on dogs which had sustained a prior myocardial infarction [36]. The animals were tested during treadmill exercise and occlusion of the left circumflex artery. When 50-60 min prior to coronary occlusion, a 70% omega-3 fatty acids concentrate was administered intravenously, fibrillation did not occur. A similar infusion of a soy bean oil emulsion resulted as expected in prompt development of ventricular fibrillation. Since the 50-60 min were too short and the administered amount not enough for raising the whole body membrane EPA and DHA content appreciably, it can be deduced that EPA and DHA present in serum had a protective action [36]. In accordance with this contention would be the finding that sustained ventricular tachycardia can be reduced by infusion of 3.8 g omega-3 marine triacylglycerols in patients with ICDs [37].

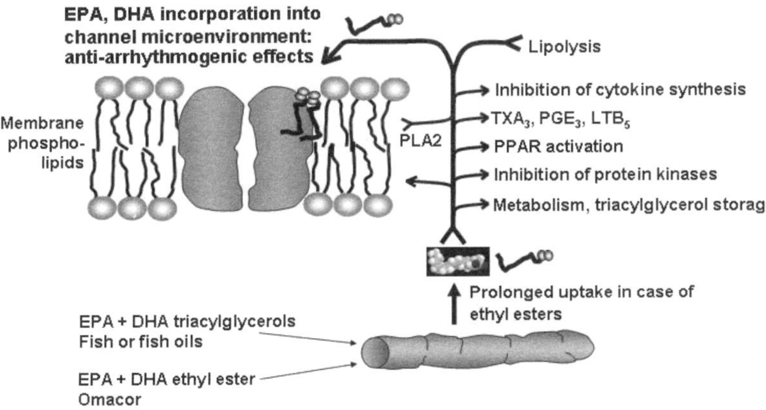

Figure 6A. Schematic representation of biological effects of EPA and DHA administered as triacylglycerols or ethyl esters. EPA attenuates some of the actions of arachidonic acid particularly via the synthesis of TXA$_3$ and LTB$_5$. The incorporation of EPA and DHA in the form of free fatty acids into the micro-environment of ion channels is based on studies of Leaf *et al* [38].

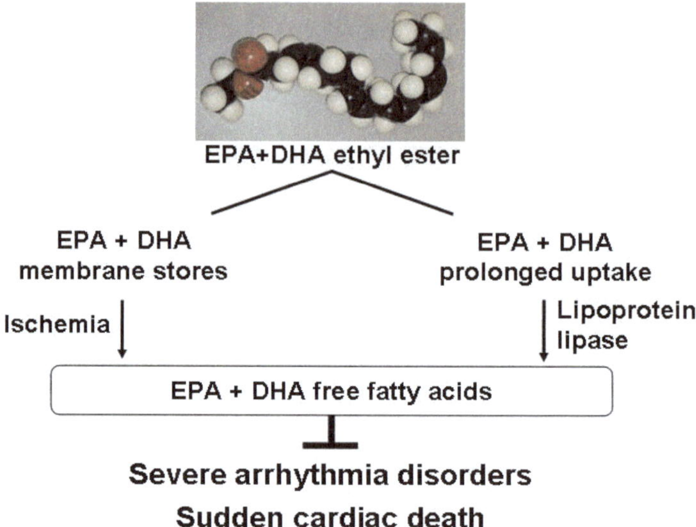

Figure 6B. Mechanisms contributing to a critical rise in EPA and DHA required for reducing the risk of severe arrhythmia disorders and sudden cardiac death. As a result of ischaemia, EPA and DHA are released from membrane phospholipids and contribute to the non-membrane bound EPA and DHA pool. In the case of ethyl ester administration, an EPA and DHA trough-to-peak ratio close to 1.0 is expected for the administration since they are absorbed in a sustained manner.

Mechanisms of Anti-arrhythmogenic Action of EPA and DHA Free Fatty Acids

In the context of our studies on effects of omega-3 fatty acids on sarcoplasmic reticulum Ca^{2+} uptake [39], cardiac hypertrophy and dilatation [40,41] and reperfusion-induced arrhythmias [42], no significant alterations in the Na^+ channel activity of papillary muscles of fish oil fed rats were found by the loose patch clamp technique [43] (Table 2). The Na^+ channel properties were not affected although the DHA content of phospholipids was increased from 9 to 28% and the number of ischaemia-reperfusion arrhythmias was reduced [42]. Thus, EPA and DHA bound to membrane phospholipids do not affect the properties of the Na^+ channel. At the time of these experiments we were not aware of findings that free fatty acids of EPA and DHA are involved in the anti-arrhythmogenic action. Free EPA and DHA were, therefore, not added during the electrophysiological experiments, which according to the later experiments of Leaf *et al* (reviewed in [38]) would have been required for observing inhibitory effects on ion channels.

Table 2. Lack of changes in steady state or kinetic parameters of the cardiac Na^+ current measured in isolated papillary muscles of rats fed 10% mackerel oil for 10-13 weeks

	Mackerel oil	Hydrogenated coconut oil	
Na^+ conductance (pS/μm^2)	159 ± 31	94 ± 8	P=0.06
Activation curves			
Hodgkin-Huxley "m" (mV)	-52 ± 2	-55 ± 1	N.S.
Steepness of "m" (mV)	11.1 ± 0.5	10.6 ± 0.4	N.S.
Steady state inactivation curve			
Midpoint (mV)	-79.7 ± 0.8	-78.4 ± 2.7	N.S.
Steepness (mV)	11.8 ± 0.8	10.2 ± 0.8	N.S.
Ischaemic zone (%)	36.8%	40.8%	N.S.
Arrhythmia incidence	0.4	3.6	P<0.05
Cardiac DHA (%)	$28.4 \pm 1.8\%$	$13.7 \pm 0.8\%$	P<0.05

In open chest rats, the left anterior descending coronary artery was constricted for 40 min. This ischaemic period was followed by 60 min reperfusion. The arrhythmia incidence was calculated summing up the total counts of arrhythmias and dividing it by the number of animals; fatty acids were determined with gas chromatography. Using the loose-patch-clamp technique no significant differences in steady state or kinetic parameters of the cardiac Na^+ current were observed [43].

In a series of detailed studies, it has been shown by Leaf *et al* that the free fatty acids of EPA and DHA but not other fatty acids inhibit the Na^+ channel activity which occurs rapidly and can be washed out [44]. In addition, the cardiac Na^+-Ca^{2+} exchanger [45] and the L-type Ca^{2+} channel [46] which has been inferred particularly in after-depolarisations were inhibited. For explaining inhibitory effects also on other channels like the transient outward K^+ current [47] and the major voltage-dependent delayed rectifier current (Kv1.5) [48] one has to infer inhibitory effects which are specific for EPA and DHA but not for a particular ion channel. Also the Ca^{2+} release from intracellular Ca^{2+} stores, the sarcoplasmic reticulum, was inhibited [49,50]. The inhibitory effects of EPA and DHA have been attributed to the non-covalent incorporation of free fatty acids into the micro-environment of ion channels and the ensuing conformational change [38] (Figure 6A). A consequence of this mechanism is that a critical concentration of free EPA and DHA has to be reached before an adequate number of channels become inhibited and anti-arrhythmogenic effects ensue. After myocardial infarction, sympathetic activity is increased due to the impaired pump performance leading to a rise in myocardial free fatty acids. The release of EPA and DHA is amplified by the preferred release of fatty acids from the inner position of phospholipids by phospholipase A2.

It might thus not be unexpected that protective effects can be smaller in patients with ICD. In contrast to ischaemic events such as myocardial infarction which raise free EPA and DHA to levels required for their anti-arrhythmogenic action, the ICD is expected to terminate re-entrant ventricular tachycardias or ventricular fibrillation before marked sympathetic activation and release of EPA and DHA occurs. In the trial by Raitt *et al* [51], 1.8 g/day EPA and DHA ethyl esters did not reduce the risk of ventricular tachycardia or ventricular fibrillation in 100 patients with ICDs when compared with 100 patients on placebo (olive oil). The Study on Omega-3 Fatty Acids and Ventricular Arrhythmia (SOFA) by Brouwer *et al* assessed effects of taking 2 g fish oil on life-threatening arrhythmias in ICD patients. At 12 months, 30% of the 273 patients in the fish oil group had experienced either life-threatening arrhythmia or death compared to 33% of the 273 patients in the placebo oil group (not statistically significant). Among the subgroup of 342 patients who previously had a myocardial infarction there was a trend towards a beneficial effect of fish oil (p=0.086). In this subgroup, 28% of the patients on fish oil experienced either life-threatening arrhythmia or death compared to 35% of the patients on placebo oil. (http://www.escardio.org/vpo/ESC_congress_information/ConferenceReleases/CPreleases/ Brouwer.htm).

Although the study appears to be underpowered for the subgroup analysis, the trend would be in accordance with the GISSI-Prevention study which included 2835 post-myocardial infarction patients in the EPA and DHA ethyl ester group. In the study by Leaf *et al* [52] 402 ICD patients were randomized to 2.6 g EPA and DHA ethyl ester or olive oil as placebo for 12 months. Compliance with the double-blind treatment was similar in the two groups; however, the non-compliance rate was high (35% of all enrollees). This might not be surprising since four 1.0 g capsules had to be taken daily. The primary end-point, time to first ICD event for ventricular tachycardia or fibrillation confirmed by stored ECG or death from any cause was borderline significant (risk reduction of 28%; p=0.057). For those who stayed on protocol for at least 11 months, the anti-arrhythmic benefit of EPA and DHA ethyl esters was improved for those with confirmed events (risk reduction of 38%; p=0.034). Why in this study capsules with only 65% EPA and DHA instead of 84% as in the case of OMACOR® were used, remains intriguing. The study again strengthens the fact that patient compliance is greatly reduced with daily four 1.0 g capsules.

Further support for anti-arrhythmogenic effects of omega-3 fatty acids was provided in the study of Calo *et al* [53]. Two 1 g capsules of EPA and DHA ethyl esters were administered during hospitalization in patients undergoing coronary artery bypass graft surgery (CABG). Postoperative atrial fibrillation developed in 27 patients of the control group (33.3%) and in 12 patients of the EPA and DHA ethyl ester group (15.2%) (p=0.013). There was no significant difference in the incidence of non-fatal postoperative complications, and postoperative mortality was similar in the EPA and DHA ethyl ester-treated patients (1.3%) versus controls (2.5%). After CABG, the EPA and DHA ethyl ester-treated patients were hospitalized for significantly fewer days than controls (7.3 ± 2.1 days vs. 8.2 ± 2.6 days, p=0.017).

In addition to inhibitory effects on ion channels by EPA and DHA, the functional impact of various putative anti-arrhythmogenic mechanisms remains to be examined in greater detail. In particular, contributions arising from an increased heart rate variability [54], an improved postischaemic recovery [55] and a reduced heart rate [56] require further attention. It remains also an intriguing possibility that the process of adverse dilatation of the heart could be attenuated by EPA and DHA as shown in the pressure overloaded rat heart. When spontaneously hypertensive rats were treated with fish oil, the degree of left ventricular hypertrophy was not affected, however, the dilatation of the left ventricle was significantly reduced (Figure 7). Since cardiac dilatation is a major predisposing factor for SCD, it could be inferred from these animal experiments that a reduced adverse geometrical remodeling of the heart contributes to the observed protection of the GISSI-Prevention study.

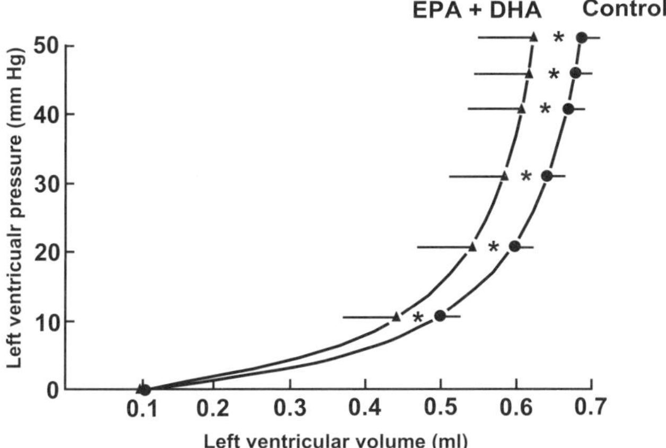

Figure 7. Attenuation of the adverse dilatation of pressure overloaded heart of spontaneously hypertensive rats by 10% fish oil feeding while the elastic material properties of the myocardium were not affected [41,57]. The passive pressure volume curve of the left ventricle is obtained by stepwise filling/emptying the arrested ventricle with defined volumes of saline. Since in the untreated rats the curve is shifted to greater volumes, it can be concluded that the omega-3 fatty acid treatment counteracted the adverse dilatation of the pressure overloaded left ventricle.

The EPA+DHA Level and the Sustained Uptake of EPA and DHA Ethyl Esters

Whether a required level of non-membrane bound EPA+DHA is reached, depends not only on the fatty acid release from tissue stores but also on the absorption of orally administered EPA and DHA. These fatty acids can be administered as the chemically prepared ethyl esters (OMACOR®), chemically prepared free fatty acids (to our knowledge not used as commercially available compounds) or the naturally occurring triacylglycerols present in fish and fish oil. Initially, the rationale for ethyl esters was to provide a high-purity EPA and DHA preparation, which reduced the number of daily required capsules. In fish, the triacylglycerols contain on average one EPA or DHA and two saturated fatty acids per glycerol molecule. Thus, in fish oils approximately one-third of the fatty acids are EPA and DHA. For achieving a much higher concentration of EPA and DHA, one has to substitute the glycerol with an alcohol with only one hydroxyl group resulting in the individual fatty acid esters. Fish oils can be transesterified with alcohol such as methanol and ethanol. Methanol is used routinely during the derivatization of fatty acids for their gas chromatographic determination. Methylation is also used for the large-scale production of plant oil based fuel ("biodiesel") [58]. In the case of omega-3 fatty acid esters for human consumption, ethanol is used which results in a mixture of saturated and unsaturated ethyl esters. Based on the different physico-chemical properties arising from chain length and number of double bonds, nearly homogeneous EPA and DHA ethyl esters can be isolated and the respective saturated fatty acids are discarded in the following purification process (Figure 8A). This procedure obviously increases the production costs when compared with the simple extraction procedure used for fish oil. An important side-effect of this purification relates to reduction in environmental pollutants such as methyl-mercury to very low levels (see below).

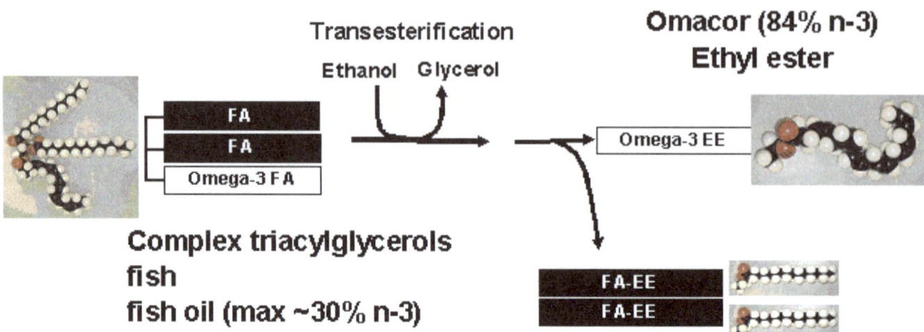

Figure 8A. Transesterification of triacylglycerols from fish leading to a highly purified EPA and DHA ethyl ester preparation. EPA and DHA are omega-3 fatty acids since the first double bond is at the position three when counting from the methyl end.

A representative gas chromatogram of OMACOR® injected directly without derivatization is shown in Figure 8B. A chromatogram is also given for a sample which was obtained by mixing 1:1 untreated OMACOR® and OMACOR® which had been transesterified with methanol. For this sample, 2 peaks corresponding to methyl and ethyl esters of EPA, DHA and other minor fatty acids were observed (Figure 8B). The procedure of transesterification has often been misinterpreted by stating that it represents just a "refinement" and ethyl esters of EPA and DHA are referred to as some kind of "highly purified fish oil" which considers, however, only one aspect of the production process. The reason why less attention has been given to the transesterification step relies probably in the fact that early comparative studies on triacylglycerols and ethyl esters have not been judged encouraging with respect to the absorption kinetics of ethyl esters. Since the GISSI-Prevention study was performed with EPA and DHA ethyl esters and a reduction in the risk of sudden death by 45% was observed, questions are raised on the biological relevance of conclusions drawn from the early studies, which judged ethyl esters as less favorable compared with triacylglycerols.

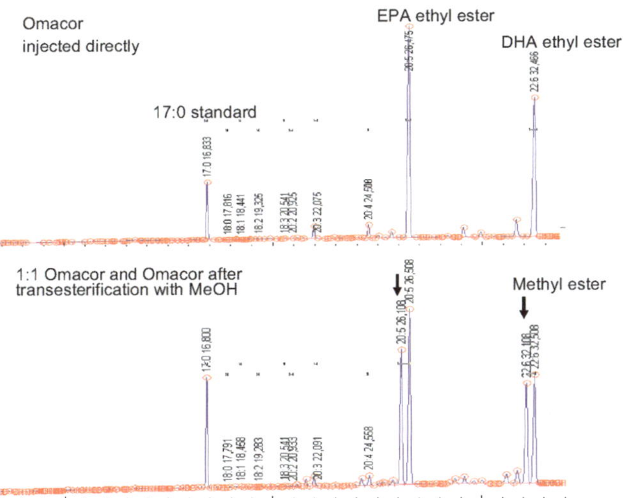

Figure 8B. A representative gas chromatogram of OMACOR® injected without derivatization into the gas chromatograph. A chromatogram is also shown for a sample which was obtained by 1:1 mixing untreated OMACOR® with OMACOR® which has been transesterified with methanol. In this sample, 2 peaks corresponding to methyl and ethyl esters of EPA, DHA and also other minor fatty acids are observed.

Lawson *et al* [59] studied in humans the plasma incorporation of EPA after administration of 1 g EPA either as ethyl ester or triacylglycerol during 8 h after intake. Ethyl esters were poorly absorbed and even triacylglycerols were not completely absorbed during this short time interval. It was concluded that ethyl esters are poor substrates for pancreatic lipase which is in accordance with *in vitro* studies. Although the absorption of ethyl esters is increased by co-ingestion with a high-fat meal, the absorption of EPA ethyl ester was still lower [60]. Also el Boustani *et al* [61] reported a reduced absorption of ethyl esters within 12 h when compared with the free fatty acid or a glycerol ester. It was, therefore, an intriguing finding by Luley *et al* [62] that in healthy volunteers the long-term (after 7-28 days) bioavailability does not differ between ethyl esters and triacylglycerols. In particular, no differences were observed after the intake of 2x 1 capsule of a 85% EPA and DHA ethyl ester preparation (1.70 g EPA+DHA) compared with 3x 2 capsules of a 32% EPA and DHA triacylglycerol preparation (1.92 g EPA+DHA). These findings are noteworthy since a twice daily administration would in general be expected to result in a lower blood level compared with a three times daily administration. Since blood was drawn in the morning and no further information is given on the time in between capsule intake and blood sampling [62], no conclusions can, however, be drawn on the peak-to-trough values of EPA and DHA concentration in the blood after the intake of EPA and DHA in the form of triacylglycerols or ethyl esters.

The type of ester bond of EPA and DHA has thus consequences for the absorption kinetics of EPA and DHA and the duodenal uptake rates differ between triacylglycerols and ethyl esters. Triacylglycerols are rapidly degraded by pancreatic lipase and, in the case of polyunsaturated fatty acids, particularly by carboxyl ester hydrolase. Compared with the corresponding triacylglycerols, the synthetic ethyl esters of EPA and DHA are absorbed more slowly. This has been shown in rats when EPA and DHA were administered by gavage either as triacylglycerols or ethyl esters and the recovery of the administered fatty acids was determined in the lymph [63]. Within 3 h after the administration, the recovery in the lymph of the respective fatty acids was greater in the case of triacylglycerols [63]

(Figure 9). After 15 h, the recovery from ethyl esters was, however, approximately doubled compared with triacylglycerols. One of the consequences is that the plasma EPA and DHA level is maintained at a higher level in the second half of a 24 h period which is of importance, since ventricular tachyarrhythmias are more abundant in the early morning hours [64]. Plasma EPA and DHA levels arising from fish consumption during the preceding day would thus be expected to be lower than in the case of an ethyl ester administration. The different absorption kinetics within a 24 h period seen in the rat appear to hold also for humans.

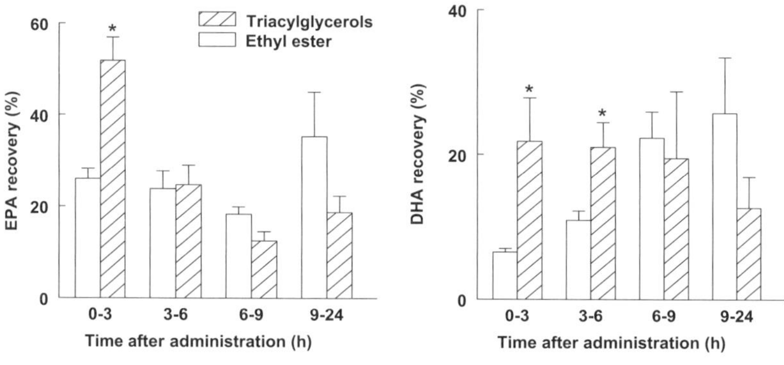

Figure 9. Recovery of EPA and DHA in the lymphe of rats administered by gavage EPA and DHA either as triacylglycerol or ethyl ester. *p<0.05 vs. ethyl esters. The total recovery after 24 h did not differ significantly between triacylglycerols and ethyl esters. Data are adapted from Ikeda *et al* [63].

We examined in healthy volunteers whether 18 h after the intake of one capsule of OMACOR®, increased concentrations of EPA and DHA occur in the serum. Concentrations were determined 18 h after intake of one capsule at days 1, 3, 7, 11, 15, 30 and 43. At day 1, 15, 30 and 43 concentrations were determined at 3, 6, 9, 18 and 24 h after the intake. EPA and DHA were increased in the serum after 3, 7, 11, 15, 30 and 43 days and the levels did not differ significantly at 3 vs. 18 h after capsule intake (H. Rupp *et al*, unpublished). These data indicate, therefore, that the "retard or slow release" formulation of ethyl esters has the advantage of providing sustained increased non-membrane bound EPA and DHA levels (in the form of blood triacylglycerols and VLDL), which are expected to contribute to the critical rise in EPA and DHA required for an anti-arrhythmogenic action.

These considerations are based on a once daily administration which is relevant in patients after myocardial infarction being on standard therapy with a beta-blocker, ACE-inhibitor, anti-platelet drug and a statin. It remains to be assessed to what extent the 45% risk reduction of sudden death observed in the GISSI-Prevention study [20,26,27] arises from the administration of ethyl esters of EPA and DHA as compared with triacylglycerols. In this respect it should be pointed out that no interventional study comparable to the GISSI-Prevention study is currently available for EPA and DHA triacylglycerols of fish or fish oils.

Dietary Sources of Omega-3 Fatty Acids

EPA and DHA triacylglycerols in prepared and frozen fish. Since in the GISSI-Prevention study 840 mg EPA and DHA ethyl esters were administered corresponding to 1 g/day OMACOR® in addition to regular fish consumption as might also be inferred from a Mediterranean lifestyle, we addressed the question to what extent dietary fish intake contributes to the desirable EPA and DHA intake. We analyzed the EPA and DHA content of fish dishes prepared at the cafeteria of the Philipps University Hospital of Marburg [24]. The most often served fish dish was Alaska pollock containing 125±70 mg/100 g EPA+DHA. In addition to EPA and DHA, fish contains the saturated fatty acids palmitic acid (C16:0), stearic acid (C18:0), the omega-9 monounsaturated fatty acid oleic acid (C18:1) and the omega-6 polyunsaturated fatty acid linoleic acid (C18:2) (Table 3). The variable content of EPA and DHA per 100 g wet weight depends on a number of factors. Omega-3 polyunsaturated fatty acids are produced by algae particularly in cold water and are taken up by fish via the food chain. It is, therefore, not unexpected that the fish Tilapia, which lives in a warm water sea, exhibits the lowest EPA and DHA content. Another influence arises from the fat content of fish as exemplified by the eel. Although the eel was caught in a river nearby Marburg, it has the highest EPA and DHA content of all fish analyzed. As expected, the locally caught non-oily/fatty fish pike exhibits a low content of EPA and DHA. From a comparison of frozen (Table 4) versus prepared (cooked/baked) fish, it can be deduced that the EPA and DHA content appears not to be reduced appreciably by the present food preparation.

Table 3. Content (mg/100g wet weight) of fatty acids in fish prepared at the cafeteria of the University Hospital (Lahnberge) Marburg

	Tilapia	Crab	Zander	Hoki	Red snapper	Pollock	Cat fish	Shell	Common sole	Eel smoked
8:0	ND	0.4	4.5	ND	ND	3.7	0.7	5.1	12.0	0.1
10:0	1.5	1.0	2.2	ND	4.0	<0.05	2.2	17.1	8.8	0.2
11:0	0.4	ND	2.2	ND	0.6	<0.05	0.3	2.2	1.0	0.3
12:0	4.0	1.6	3.4	ND	7.9	0.5	3.7	23.8	16.6	5.5
13:0	0.5	ND	1.0	ND	0.4	<0.05	0.3	ND	2.5	<0.05
14:0	53.4	6.6	15.0	3.6	27.6	10.8	26.3	109.8	73.0	147.0
14:1	3.6	0.4	2.7	ND	1.6	0.2	1.5	4.5	0.8	4.5
15:0	5.3	2.7	5.0	0.8	4.3	1.1	4.1	20.8	13.2	13.2
15:1	0.1	<0.05	0.5	<0.05	ND	ND	<0.05	0.2	<0.05	0.3
16:0	395.2	54.0	133.6	156.1	170.0	353.4	159.5	443.4	306.7	748.9
16:1	70.7	6.9	11.0	9.8	19.1	4.9	48.1	109.7	67.8	354.3
17:1	ND	ND	3.5	ND	ND	8.9	0.6	2.8	7.7	11.8
18:0	99.0	22.3	36.3	34.6	54.7	50.5	39.7	117.0	91.8	148.9
18:1n9t	9.1	0.4	3.8	0.4	3.1	2.5	4.6	6.2	16.7	3.9
18:1n9c	478.1	18.8	169.6	93.5	102.9	438.4	175.6	173.9	198.1	947.1
18:2n6t	<0.05	0.1	1.0	ND	0.2	<0.05	0.2	ND	0.2	6.2
18:2n6c	234.5	2.4	101.1	10.7	14.5	117.0	13.0	34.6	17.1	98.1
20:0	3.7	0.2	4.1	ND	0.5	3.8	0.4	1.5	1.4	3.0
18:3n6	10.8	0.1	1.3	ND	0.8	0.4	0.3	0.8	9.8	2.7
20:1	22.9	0.7	5.9	3.4	1.9	6.8	50.6	34.2	7.6	23.3
18:3n3	16.4	1.0	5.1	1.6	3.2	0.7	9.4	38.0	6.1	88.1
21:0	0.6	<0.05	23.7	ND	0.2	12.2	2.6	20.5	4.0	0.7
20:2	13.9	1.1	1.1	0.8	1.2	0.2	5.5	25.7	6.3	14.0
20:3n9	ND	ND	ND	ND	ND	ND	ND	ND	ND	0.6
22:0	1.2	0.3	2.4	ND	0.6	0.6	0.3	0.4	ND	0.7
20:3n6	13.4	0.6	0.6	0.4	2.1	0.6	0.5	2.0	17.4	7.3
22:1n9	1.0	3.9	1.0	0.2	0.5	1.4	2.5	0.5	4.6	0.9
20:3n3	2.4	0.4	4.0	0.1	0.6	0.5	ND	1.6	3.8	9.3
20:4n6	28.9	7.9	20.6	14.3	40.3	8.2	31.7	19.3	77.7	46.1
23:0	ND	ND	0.1	ND	0.2	ND	0.1	2.0	ND	1.5
22:2	ND	ND	2.2	ND	ND	2.0	0.3	3.4	12.4	12.1
24:0	2.7	ND	1.6	ND	ND	<0.05	ND	ND	0.9	ND
20:5n3	1.9	42.9	28.0	44.2	18.8	58.2	85.2	174.6	55.7	115.4
24:1	ND	ND	5.9	1.0	1.2	1.1	ND	0.1	ND	0.6
22:6n3	15.5	23.0	81.5	188.1	124.6	119.2	136.7	223.6	286.4	103.4
EPA+DHA	17.4	66.0	109.5	232.3	143.3	177.4	222.0	398.1	342.1	218.9

Table 4. Content (mg/100g wet weight) of fatty acids in frozen fish

	Cod	Plaice	Pollock	Alaska Pollock	"wild" Pollock	Pike	Eel
8:0	ND	ND	1.2	0.7	ND	14.9	9.5
10:0	ND	ND	0.1	<0.05	0.2	4.3	0.1
11:0	ND	ND	<0.05	<0.05	0.3	0.7	2.7
12:0	ND	ND	0.3	0.2	0.9	1.9	18.3
13:0	ND	ND	<0.05	<0.05	0.1	3.1	1.5
14:0	4.1	21.9	1.4	0.9	25.7	2.7	200.8
14:1	ND	1.4	<0.05	<0.05	0.2	2.8	7.0
15:0	1.2	4.9	0.5	0.2	2.4	3.1	27.1
15:1	0.1	1.4	<0.05	<0.05	<0.05	3.0	2.3
16:0	80.3	154.9	31.0	29.1	90.5	52.0	1026.0
16:1	ND	76.8	1.1	1.6	22.2	9.2	627.7
17:1	0.8	3.9	0.3	0.1	2.4	2.7	33.0
18:0	14.5	24.8	8.9	4.7	46.8	18.7	203.3
18:1n9t	<0.05	8.2	0.3	0.2	ND	2.0	20.6
18:1n9c	50.1	105.5	20.6	10.9	136.9	30.3	1999.3
18:2n6t	1.2	3.9	<0.05	<0.05	3.4	1.4	10.1
18:2n6c	2.3	6.2	1.9	5.2	9.0	11.7	163.1
20:0	0.2	0.8	0.1	0.2	5.2	10.1	42.1
18:3n6	1.5	3.9	2.0	3.8	0.1	3.5	41.9
20:1	0.7	9.3	6.6	0.8	74.2	3.7	53.3
18:3n3	2.2	9.2	<0.05	ND	11.5	1.2	48.9
21:0	1.1	1.7	0.7	0.5	0.4	3.4	172.3
20:2	0.9	3.7	0.3	0.1	4.0	3.9	63.6
20:3n9	ND	ND	ND	ND	0.4	ND	ND
22:0	0.8	1.2	<0.05	<0.05	0.4	0.1	24.8
20:3n6	1.2	1.6	2.1	1.8	1.0	5.8	28.5
22:1n9	1.4	0.3	0.3	0.2	ND	2.0	6.6
20:3n3	0.4	0.1	<0.05	<0.05	ND	5.2	7.6
20:4n6	8.0	23.6	2.7	1.0	45.5	22.9	86.8
23:0	3.3	0.1	ND	ND	1.6	ND	ND
22:2	1.0	1.7	ND	<0.05	5.8	8.0	4.2
24:0	0.2	0.1	0.7	0.3	0.1	6.2	53.2
20:5n3	36.1	112.4	10.8	12.1	52.7	24.3	292.1
24:1	ND	0.3	1.8	0.7	2.5	7.1	6.3
22:6n3	129.2	24.1	55.5	37.2	166.1	95.3	155.0
EPA+DHA	165.3	186.5	66.3	49.3	218.8	119.6	447.1

Taking into account that the average daily fish intake in Northern Germany is 18 g and 13 g in Southern Germany [65], it can be concluded that the dietary fish intake is too low for providing 840 mg EPA and DHA per day. This conclusion holds also for the Eastern part of Germany with 19 g/day fish consumption [66]. Fish consumption in Germany appears to be comparable to that reported in the GISSI-Prevention study where at the beginning of the study 73.2% consumed once per week fish and 87.6% at the end [20,26,27].

Although fish consumption cannot provide the EPA and DHA intake achieved in the GISSI-Prevention study, it appears to have various beneficial effects in primary prevention as demonstrated in epidemiological studies. Mortality from coronary heart disease was lower among those who consumed at least 30 g of fish per day than among those who did not eat fish [67]. Among adults, modest consumption of tuna or other broiled or baked fish, but not fried fish or fish sandwiches, was associated with lower mortality risk of ischaemic heart disease, especially arrhythmic death [68]. In a prospective study in diabetic women, an inverse association between fish and long-chain omega-3 fatty acid consumption and risk of coronary heart disease and total mortality was observed [69]. A recent meta-analysis of 11 studies including 222,364 individuals with an average 11.8 years of follow-up showed that, compared with those who never consumed fish or ate fish less than once per month, individuals with a higher intake of fish had lower coronary heart disease mortality [70]. However, in intervention trials involving intake of EPA and DHA triacylglycerols, cardiovascular effects were far less pronounced. Thus, 6 g/day of EPA and DHA triacylglycerols for 3 months followed by 3 g/day for 21 months only modestly mitigated the course of coronary atherosclerosis [71].

Based on the current evidence derived from epidemiological and interventional studies, it was pointed out in a scientific statement of the American Heart Association that patients with documented coronary heart disease should consume approximately 1 g/day EPA and DHA while subjects without documented coronary heart disease should eat (preferably) oily fish at least twice a week [72]. This recommendation is wider than the current indication for OMACOR®, which is a prescription drug in Germany for post-myocardial infarction patients in addition to standard therapy. In the guidelines of the European Society of Cardiology for the management of ST elevation myocardial infarction, supplementation with 1 g fish oil omega-3 polyunsaturated fatty acids was rated as class I recommendation, level of evidence B (because of currently only one randomized study, i.e. GISSI-Prevention study) [73].

EPA and DHA triacylglycerols in fish oils. To compare the intake of EPA and DHA triacylglycerols from fish dishes with that of fish oils, we analyzed the EPA and DHA content of 11 over-the-counter brands of fish oil capsules available in Germany. Using the C17:0 fatty acid standard, the amount of EPA and DHA per capsule was determined and compared with the specified content. The capsules differed markedly with respect to their EPA and DHA content per capsule (Table 5). The EPA and DHA content calculated for 1 g capsule content was comparable within the brands containing oil from pollock approaching 300 mg/g EPA and DHA [24]. This might suggest that the fish oils used for producing the capsules were similar, however, the oils differed actually with respect to the composition of other fatty acids. Major fatty acids were the saturated fatty acids palmitic acid (C16:0), stearic acid (C18:0), oleic acid (C18:1) and arachidonic acid (C20:4) reflecting the composition of fish. Liver oils from halibut and cod are characterized by greater amounts of oleic acid and alpha-linolenic acid. In contrast to cod liver oil, the halibut oil capsules contained only a small amount of EPA and DHA.

Table 5. Fatty acid content (mg per capsule) of 11 over-the-counter fish oil brands (labeled as of Pollock origin), halibut liver oil, cod liver oil and OMACOR®

	Fish oil 1	Fish oil 2	Fish oil 3	Fish oil 4	Fish oil 5	Fish oil 6	Fish oil 7	Fish oil 8	Fish oil 9	Fish oil 10	Fish oil 11	Halibut liver oil	Cod liver oil	Omacor
8:0	0.2	ND	ND	ND	ND	ND	ND	ND	ND	ND	ND	ND	ND	1.4
10:0	<0.05	<0.05	1.5	0.1	0.1	ND	ND	ND	ND	ND	ND	ND	<0.05	0.8
11:0	<0.05	<0.05	<0.05	<0.05	<0.05	ND	ND	ND	ND	ND	ND	ND	0.1	0.1
12:0	1.1	0.7	1.3	0.7	0.5	ND	ND	ND	ND	ND	ND	ND	0.5	0.4
13:0	0.4	0.2	0.4	0.2	0.2	ND	ND	ND	ND	ND	ND	ND	0.3	<0.05
14:0	66.3	32.6	62.1	34.9	34.4	38.4	40.7	49.7	27.7	65.3	90.9	1.4	66.6	0.3
14:1	0.3	0.5	0.3	0.3	0.1	0.3	0.3	0.5	0.3	0.6	0.8	<0.05	1.6	0.1
15:0	4.7	2.3	4.8	3.3	2.4	3.1	3.2	3.2	1.9	4.4	5.9	0.2	5.9	0.1
15:1	0.1	<0.05	0.2	0.4	0.3	<0.05	0.4	0.1	<0.05	<0.05	0.1	<0.05	1.0	0.2
16:0	136.2	73.9	143.3	79.8	75.2	92.1	87.1	119.2	54.2	160.3	178.0	17.0	203.0	0.4
16:1	73.4	35.6	75.2	36.8	42.8	46.4	47.4	49.3	28.4	70.0	94.3	2.4	142.0	1.4
17:1	10.0	3.9	10.2	4.7	6.0	7.1	6.7	7.8	5.1	11.0	15.4	0.2	17.6	<0.05
18:0	26.3	13.0	26.3	16.3	15.8	25.7	22.4	44.8	16.1	64.3	46.6	5.1	27.6	0.7
18:1n9t	1.2	0.6	11.8	4.9	6.6	0.8	0.5	1.0	0.4	0.9	1.9	0.1	53.9	0.2
18:1n9c	71.3	44.6	84.8	56.3	57.6	73.8	45.1	67.7	32.8	62.2	91.0	182.0	432.1	1.2
18:2n6t	0.7	0.2	2.7	1.9	0.8	9.2	0.6	ND	0.4	1.0	1.3	0.3	3.8	<0.05
18:2n6c	29.8	10.0	17.2	6.1	8.6	16.5	6.7	7.4	3.7	10.9	14.2	54.8	28.0	1.2
20:0	9.9	1.3	1.2	1.0	1.1	1.2	1.3	2.0	0.8	2.3	2.8	1.7	2.3	0.3
18:3n6	3.3	0.8	4.6	0.6	1.5	1.0	1.5	1.2	0.7	2.4	2.2	1.7	3.9	ND
20:1	9.3	1.6	14.1	11.0	10.4	1.6	0.5	0.8	0.6	1.1	1.5	1.7	ND	1.0
18:3n3	8.8	11.5	10.8	3.4	1.2	5.2	4.4	5.7	2.5	6.2	9.1	24.1	234.9	0.4
21:0	0.4	0.1	1.3	0.3	0.7	1.3	ND	ND	ND	ND	ND	ND	ND	ND
20:2	24.0	0.9	30.0	17.2	11.8	13.3	17.6	19.4	8.9	23.5	35.5	5.8	ND	16.2
20:3n9	4.1	12.2	0.6	0.6	0.4	ND	1.3	ND	ND	ND	ND	ND	ND	ND
22:0	1.4	0.6	1.1	0.3	0.2	0.2	0.2	0.2	0.2	0.4	0.3	0.1	ND	5.5
20:3n6	1.7	0.5	2.7	1.2	0.7	0.3	0.8	0.9	ND	1.0	1.5	0.9	ND	1.1
22:1n9	5.3	8.7	ND	ND	ND	0.5	0.5	0.1	ND	0.1	0.1	0.1	ND	0.3
20:3n3	1.3	0.7	ND	2.0	4.9	0.3	0.4	0.6	0.7	0.7	0.9	<0.05	ND	0.2
20:4n6	6.8	3.0	22.4	6.1	5.2	4.8	5.2	6.1	4.5	7.6	11.9	1.8	165.5	29.0
23:0	ND	ND	0.5	0.9	0.2	<0.05	ND	ND	0.1	0.1	0.1	1.5	12.3	ND
22:2	0.3	3.9	9.2	ND	ND	5.9	4.5	4.4	2.4	6.9	8.8	0.3	ND	0.3
24:0	0.1	<0.05	ND	ND	ND	0.5	0.2	<0.05	0.1	<0.05	0.2	<0.05	ND	2.8
20:5n3	147.8	58.3	140.4	63.7	67.7	65.0	87.0	98.8	55.9	120.0	173.6	1.4	175.9	490.8
24:1	<0.05	1.8	4.8	ND	ND	<0.05	<0.05	<0.05	<0.05	<0.05	<0.05	<0.05	3.4	9.2
22:6n3	101.1	40.4	87.4	67.1	43.3	58.6	59.3	60.5	33.0	80.0	102.0	1.5	207.8	391.4
Capsule content (mg)	991	499	845	502	498	498	501	544	299	680	980	275	1000	996
EPA+DHA	248.9	98.7	227.8	130.7	111.0	123.6	146.3	159.3	88.9	200.0	275.6	2.9	383.8	882
specified EPA+DHA	297.4	120	255	150 n3	150 n3	120	NA	150 n3	NA	180 n3	309 n3	NA	NA	840

Note, the high content of EPA and DHA in Omacor as compared with fish oils. When presently unidentified fatty acids were included in the area integration of Omacor, the EPA concentration was reduced from 51.3% to 45.6% and DHA from 40.9% to 36.3%. The content per capsule was not affected.

Mercury, dioxins and PCBs in fish products. One might argue that the amount of daily consumed fish or fish oil could be raised in general. A problem associated with a high intake of fish relates to the contamination with methyl-mercury and various environmental pollutants including dioxins and polychlorinated biphenyls (PCBs). According to the US Environmental Protection Agency, the maximum safe level of mercury in edible fish is 0.55 ppm which was exceeded in a recent study in 4 out of 5 fish in California waters, whereby the maximum content was 7.5 ppm [74]. It is, therefore, not unexpected that patients in San Francisco with a history of fish consumption had a mercury blood level of 15 µg/l (women) and 13 µg/l (men) [75] which correspond to 0.015 and 0.013 ppm. The mean level for women in this survey was 10 times that of mercury levels found in a recent population survey by the U.S. Centers for Disease Control and Prevention. Some children were >40 times the national mean. Mercury levels declined after stopping fish consumption. Although symptoms of mercury poisoning apparently arising from consuming tuna steak almost every night were observed as having trouble concentrating, feeling sluggish and experiencing hand tremors, they appear not to be experienced by all subjects [76]. In preschool Inuit children from Canada, tremor amplitude was related to blood mercury concentrations, which corroborates an effect already reported among adults [77]. In accordance, the Food and Drug Administration advised pregnant women and children not to exceed 3 to 4 fish servings per week and to avoid certain predatory fish [72].

Although PCBs have various negative health consequences [76], specific adverse actions on the cardiovascular system have been reported for mercury. The mercury level in the toenail which represents a long-term storage site for heavy metals was directly associated with the risk of myocardial infarction while, as expected, the adipose-tissue DHA level was inversely associated with the risk [78]. After adjustment for the DHA level and coronary risk factors, the mercury levels in patients were 15% higher than those in controls. The risk-factor-adjusted odds ratio for myocardial infarction associated with the highest as compared with the lowest quintile of mercury was 2.16 (P for trend=0.006). After adjustment for the mercury level, the DHA level was inversely associated with the risk of myocardial infarction (P for trend=0.02). A high mercury content may, therefore, diminish the cardioprotective effect of fish intake. It was concluded that substitution of fish with high methyl-mercury concentrations with fish containing less methyl-mercury among women of childbearing age yield substantial developmental benefits and few negative impacts [79]. If women instead decrease fish consumption, countervailing risks substantially reduce net benefits. If other adults reduce their fish consumption, the net public health impact is expected to be negative [79].

The question arises, therefore, whether fish oil capsules provide a substitute of fish intake in primary prevention with the suggested two fish meals per week. The mercury content of 3 over-the-counter fish oil supplements was <6 µg/l, in one brand 10 µg/l and in another brand 12 µg/l [80]. In fish oils, the amount of PCBs and organochlorine pesticides was less than the Food and Drug Administration daily recommended limits [80]. However, in an extensive study of the UK Food Standards Agency, in 12 of the 33 samples of fish oil supplements, the concentration of dioxins exceeded the European Commission's limit for dioxins which compares with 10 out of 15 samples in an Irish study (http://www.food.gov.uk/multimedia/pdfs/26diox.pdf). Manufacturers were asked to withdraw batches of two products which, on their own, could result in intakes of dioxins and dioxin like PCBs that would exceed twice the Tolerable Daily Intake (TDI). While not stated in guidelines, it appears that patients with coronary heart disease should have a much lower intake of toxins particularly mercury since they have been advised to consume 1 g EPA and DHA per day. In particular, a daily 1 g EPA and DHA dosage is advised for post-myocardial infarction patients who have already a markedly increased risk for coronary events. EPA and DHA supplements for post-myocardial infarction patients should, therefore, have toxin levels which are as low as technically achievable. For minimizing the amount of methyl-mercury and other lipid soluble environmental toxins, various purification steps including the transesterification procedure appear to be needed. While over-the-counter dietary supplements are currently not obliged to specify the content of mercury and other toxins, it is suggested to include the mercury level specification and the low abundance of other toxins on the package for EPA and DHA preparations available at prescription. Also by this way, the distinction between dietary supplements used as replacement for fish meals and a prescription drug for secondary prevention in post-myocardial infarction patients would become more readily apparent.

Endogenous Production of EPA and DHA from Alpha-Linolenic Acid

It has been argued that the short-chain omega-3 fatty acid alpha-linolenic acid derived from plants could be consumed for increasing the amount of EPA and DHA in the body by the enzymes Δ-6 desaturase and Δ-5 desaturase (Figure 10). Of particular interest are plant oils with a high proportion of alpha-linolenic acid such as linseed oil, canola oil/rapeseed oil and walnut oil (Table 6). For the rat we have shown that feeding increasingly greater amounts of linseed oil does not increase the content of EPA and DHA in the aorta [81] (Table 7). However, the enhanced alpha-linolenic acid intake reduced the arachidonic acid level and enhanced the production of PGF_{1alpha} which is the stable degradation product of prostacyclin. Thus, although an increased alpha-linolenic acid intake did not raise the EPA+DHA level, it resulted in an enhanced production of prostacyclin which, in addition to various cytoprotective actions, is a potent inhibitor of platelet aggregation. The increased prostacyclin production is expected to contribute to the improvement in endothelial function when the alpha-linolenic intake is increased [82].

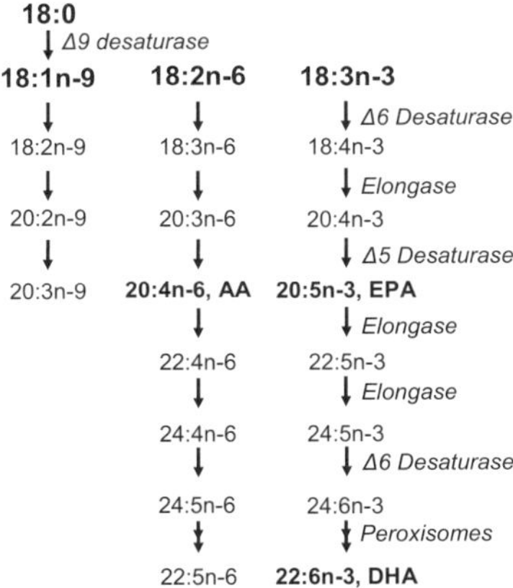

Figure 10. Biosynthesis of unsaturated fatty acids. Oleic acid (18:1n-9) can be produced by humans while linoleic acid (18:2n-6) and linolenic acid (18:3n-6) are essential fatty acids and are produced mainly by plants. EPA and DHA are produced by marine algae which are taken up by fish via the food chain. When referring to an "omega-3 level", one has to include also the short-chain omega-3 fatty acid alpha-linolenic acid as well as the long-chain omega-3 fatty acids EPA and DHA. When 24:5n-6 (6,9,12,15,18-24:5) and 24:6n-3 (6,9,12,15,18,21-24:6) are produced in the endoplasmic reticulum, they move to peroxisomes for conversion to 22:5n-6 (4,7,10,13,16-22:5) and 22:6n-3 (4,7,10,13,16,19-22:6) [83].

Table 6. Fatty acid composition (%) of plant oils as potential sources of alpha-linolenic acid which is the precursor fatty acid of EPA and DHA.

	Linseed oil	Canola/rape seed oil	Walnut	Sunflower oil	Olive oil	Perilla oil
8:0	ND	ND	<0.05	ND	ND	<0.05
10:0	<0.05	<0.05	<0.05	<0.05	<0.05	0.1
11:0	<0.05	<0.05	<0.05	<0.05	<0.05	<0.05
12:0	<0.05	<0.05	<0.05	<0.05	<0.05	<0.05
13:0	<0.05	<0.05	<0.05	<0.05	<0.05	<0.05
14:0	<0.05	0.1	<0.05	0.1	<0.05	<0.05
14:1	<0.05	<0.05	<0.05	<0.05	<0.05	<0.05
15:0	<0.05	<0.05	<0.05	<0.05	<0.05	<0.05
15:1	<0.05	ND	<0.05	<0.05	<0.05	<0.05
16:0	5.3	4.6	7.5	6.4	12.5	13.6
16:1	0.1	0.2	0.2	0.1	0.9	0.2
17:1	ND	<0.05	<0.05	<0.05	0.1	<0.05
18:0	1.2	0.7	3.9	4.6	1.5	1.6
18:1n9t	8.9	ND	ND	<0.05	ND	<0.05
18:1n9c	13.0	64.6	15.2	30.0	77.4	14.3
18:2n6t	2.9	0.5	ND	ND	ND	<0.05
18:2n6c	12.0	19.9	59.3	55.8	5.5	12.8
20:0	ND	0.7	0.4	1.5	0.8	0.1
18:3n6	ND	0.2	0.3	ND	ND	0.1
20:1	ND	ND	6.5	0.1	ND	ND
18:3n3	56.1	8.0	6.5	0.5	1.0	56.6
21:0	ND	ND	0.2	<0.05	0.1	ND
20:2	0.2	0.1	0.1	<0.05	<0.05	0.2
20:3n9	0.2	0.3	<0.05	0.5	0.1	0.2
22:0	<0.05	ND	<0.05	<0.05	<0.05	ND
20:3n6	<0.05	<0.05	<0.05	<0.05	<0.05	<0.05
22:1n9	<0.05	ND	<0.05	0.1	ND	<0.05
20:3n3	<0.05	<0.05	<0.05	<0.05	0.1	<0.05
20:4n6	<0.05	<0.05	<0.05	<0.05	<0.05	<0.05
23:0	<0.05	<0.05	<0.05	<0.05	<0.05	<0.05
22:2	ND	0.2	<0.05	<0.05	<0.05	<0.05
24:0	<0.05	ND	<0.05	0.2	<0.05	<0.05
20:5n3	<0.05	<0.05	<0.05	<0.05	<0.05	<0.05
24:1	<0.05	<0.05	<0.05	<0.05	<0.05	<0.05
22:6n3	<0.05	<0.05	<0.05	0.1	<0.05	<0.05

Table 7. Effect of an increased dietary alpha-linolenic acid intake on the fatty acid composition and prostanoids of the aorta of spontaneously hypertensive rats

	Control	1%	2.5%	5%
18:3n3	2.3 ± 0.6	4.7 ± 1.6*	7.6 ± 0.9*	11.7 ± 2.2*
20:4n6	14.4 ± 3.4	12.2 ± 2.5	11.8 ± 3.6	10.4 ± 3.1*
20:5n3	0.2 ± 0.2	0.1 ± 0.1	0.3 ± 0.2	0.4 ± 0.3
22:6n3	1.5 ± 0.5	1.4 ± 0.8	1.4 ± 0.5	0.6 ± 0.2
N6/n3	6.4 ± 1.3	4.7 ± 1.1*	3.1 ± 0.3*	2.3 ± 0.2*
PGF_{1alpha}	1.0 ± 0.3	1.8 ± 0.8	3.6 ± 1.8*	5.1 ± 1.4*

Rats were fed diets containing 1%, 2.5% and 5% linseed oil for 15-16 weeks. Prostanoids were determined with HPLC and electrochemical detection (as 2,4-dimethoxyanilides after derivatization). TXB_2, PGE_2 and PGF_{2alpha} were not altered. Systolic and diastolic blood pressure measured by radio telemetry was reduced by 6 mm Hg (in sleeping phase) after 5% linseed oil feeding for 7 weeks. Data are from Rupp *et al* [81].

A further beneficial action of polyunsaturated fatty acids relates to their triacylglycerol-lowering. As shown in rat experiments, a correlation exists between the serum triacylglycerol and free fatty acid concentration and the unsaturation index of fatty acids [39] (Figure 11). For omega-3 fatty acids, additional specific actions have to be inferred. EPA but not DHA inhibited the diacylglycerol acyltransferase, thereby reducing the biosynthesis of triacylglycerols [84]. If intracellular EPA becomes elevated it is expected to activate PPARalpha which is a major determinant for the gene expression of enzymes involved in fatty acid oxidation. PPARalpha is down regulated in failing heart [85] and by this mechanism also the fatty acid profile is expected to be altered (Rupp *et al*, unpublished).

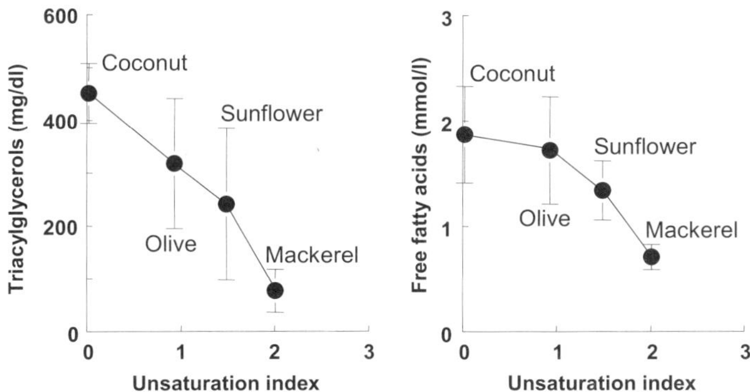

Figure 11. The inter-relationship between the serum concentration of triacylglycerols or free fatty acids and the unsaturation index in rats fed 6 weeks diets which contained 10% coconut fat, 10% olive oil, 10% sunflower oil or 10% mackerel oil. The unsaturation index was calculated by multiplying the percent proportion of each fatty acid with the number of double bonds contained in that fatty acid. The values thus obtained were summed over all the fatty acids present. The average number of double bonds per molecule was obtained by referring the number of double bonds to 100%. Data are adapted from Rupp *et al* [39].

In humans with a background diet high in saturated fat, the conversion rate of alpha-linolenic acid was found to be 6% for EPA and 3.8% for DHA [86]. However, with a diet rich in omega-6 polyunsaturated fatty acids, conversion was reduced by 40 to 50% [86]. In women of reproductive age, an increased conversion of alpha-linolenic acid into EPA (21%) and DHA (9%) was found which is higher than in men [87]. The higher conversion capacity appears to be important for meeting the demands of the fetus and neonate during pregnancy and lactation [87]. In this respect it is of great interest that any administered DHA can be retroconverted to EPA [88]. As regards secondary prevention of myocardial infarction, alpha-linolenic acid cannot be converted into amounts of EPA and DHA which have been used in the GISSI-Prevention study [20,26,27]. There is also increasing evidence that the capacity for EPA and DHA production becomes reduced in patients with cardiac dysfunction (Rupp *et al*, unpublished).

It is of particular interest to compare the risk reduction by omega-3 fatty acids and established prescription drugs in patients with coronary heart disease as done in a recent meta-analysis on antilipidemic interventions including 97 studies with 137,140 individuals in intervention and 138,976 individuals in control groups [89]. Compared with control groups, risk ratios for overall mortality were 0.87 for statins, 1.00 for fibrates, 0.84 for resins, 0.96 for niacin, 0.77 for omega-3 fatty acids, and 0.97 for diet [89]. The mortality risk was reduced significantly only by statins and omega-3 fatty acids. Although this meta-analysis included also presumable effects of alpha-linolenic acid, a major contribution is expected to arise from EPA and DHA. Also based on the evaluation of primary and secondary prevention studies, it was concluded that the "Omega-3 Index" (red blood cell EPA+DHA) may represent a novel, physiologically relevant, easily modified, independent, and graded risk factor for death from coronary heart disease that could have significant clinical utility [90].

Conclusion

Taken together, there is increasing evidence that omega-3 fatty acids exhibit various protective actions in the cardiovascular system. A protection has been inferred from primary prevention studies based on the intake of fish. Stronger evidence comes from interventional studies with EPA and DHA ethyl ester administration involving post-myocardial infarction patients [20] and ICD patients [52]. Best characterized is currently the link between a low EPA+DHA level and the risk for SCD. Based on the studies of Albert *et al* [25] and Siscovick *et al* [29] demonstrating a markedly reduced risk of SCD in persons who exhibit about 3% more EPA and DHA compared with the quartile with the lowest EPA+DHA level, it appears that about 6% blood EPA+DHA represents a target level for prevention of SCD (Figure 6). This target level is based also on our own data showing that 1 g/day OMACOR® raises the EPA+DHA level from 3.5 to 5.7% of total fatty acids. The 1 g/day OMACOR® dose equals the regimen of the GISSI-Prevention study where the risk of total mortality, cardiovascular mortality and sudden death was significantly reduced [20,26,27]. It appears, however, that an upper limit of EPA and DHA concentrations exists above which further coronary heart disease benefit may not occur [30]. This seems to be the case with the 6.2-7.4% range of EPA+DHA in serum phospholipids since an increase to 10.3% by administering 4 g/day OMACOR® had no further significant effect on the prognosis of cardiac events despite significant triacylglycerol-lowering [91]. This intriguing study by Nilsen *et al* was performed in Norway where the baseline EPA+DHA level was much higher than in other countries [30] including our own data. Whether adverse effects of mercury intake arising from fish might have interfered with protective actions of EPA and DHA remains unresolved.

In addition to the levels of incorporated EPA and DHA, one should take into account that the type of ester of administered EPA and DHA is of functional relevance. Compared with triacylglycerols present in fish and fish oils, OMACOR® contains ethyl esters which provide a prolonged uptake. Taking into account that anti-arrhythmogenic effects appear to require the free fatty acids EPA and DHA, a therapeutic intervention which provides a sustained increase in plasma EPA and DHA levels should be advantageous. An ethyl ester preparation has also the advantage of only one capsule per day. As exemplified in the study of Leaf *et al* [52], the non-compliance rate is increased to 35% of ICD patients on four 1 g capsules per day.

Clearly, further work is required to delineate the relevance of other fatty acids [92] mentioned only briefly in the present overview. One should also try to dissect protective actions which are common for EPA and DHA and selective effects of EPA and DHA. In this respect, terms such as "omega-3 level" are inaccurate when referring to EPA+DHA, since it has to include by definition the short-chain omega-3 alpha-linolenic acid as well as the long-chain EPA and DHA. As shown in rats fed increasing amounts of alpha-linolenic acid, the "omega-3 level" was increased due to the incorporation of alpha-linolenic acid while the EPA+DHA level was not altered [81]. Furthermore, the term "omega-3 level" has to include docosapentaenoic acid which was, however, not predictive of SCD in the study of Albert *et al* [25].

In view of the present evidence, it is suggested to include the determination of fatty acid profile in the list of investigated parameters, particularly in patients after myocardial infarction. This would strengthen the rationale of therapeutic regimens with EPA and DHA as specified in current guidelines [72,73]. Since only 10 µl of whole blood are required for the determination of a profile involving more than 35 fatty acids, it does rarely require additional blood sampling. By monitoring the EPA+DHA level, patients could be identified who are at an increased risk of SCD irrespective of their underlying disease. Of particular relevance would be the determination in patients with a reduced ejection fraction who exhibited a greater risk reduction with the administration of OMACOR® in the GISSI-Prevention study [93]. Furthermore, longitudinal changes in the EPA and DHA incorporation can be monitored and it can be assessed whether a required EPA+DHA level has been reached in a particular patient. Further work is required to assess to what extent the protection associated with a given whole blood EPA+DHA level is influenced by the pathophysiology of severe arrhythmia disorders. In particular, to what extent differences occur between re-entry tachyarrhythmias in the absence of a severe ischaemic event and tachyarrhythmias arising from myocardial infarction linked with sympathetic nervous system activation and release of polyunsaturated fatty acids.

References

[1]　S.S. Chugh, J. Jui, K. Gunson *et al.* Current burden of sudden cardiac death: multiple source surveillance versus retrospective death certificate-based review in a large U.S. community. *J. Am. Coll. Cardiol.* **44** (2004) 1268-1275.

[2]　N. Frasure-Smith, F. Lespérance, M. Talajic. Depression and 18-month prognosis after myocardial infarction. *Circulation* **91** (1995) 999-1005.

[3]　Y. Osher, Y. Bersudsky, R.H. Belmaker. Omega-3 eicosapentaenoic acid in bipolar depression: report of a small open-label study. *J. Clin. Psychiatry* **66** (2005) 726-729.

[4]　M.T. Kearney, K.A. Fox, A.J. Lee *et al.* Predicting sudden death in patients with mild to moderate chronic heart failure. *Heart* **90** (2004) 1137-1143.

[5]　C.G. Brilla, R.C. Funck, H. Rupp. Lisinopril-mediated regression of myocardial fibrosis in patients with hypertensive heart disease. *Circulation* **102** (2000) 1388-1393.

[6]   C.G. Brilla, H. Rupp, B. Maisch. Effects of ACE inhibition versus non-ACE inhibitor antihypertensive treatment on myocardial fibrosis in patients with arterial hypertension. Retrospective analysis of 120 patients with left ventricular endomyocardial biopsies. *Herz* **28** (2003) 744-753.

[7]   M. Turcani and H. Rupp. Etomoxir improves left ventricular performance of pressure-overloaded rat heart. *Circulation* **96** (1997) 3681-3686.

[8]   H. Rupp, W. Schulze, R. Vetter. Dietary medium-chain triglycerides can prevent changes in myosin and SR due to CPT-1 inhibition by etomoxir. *Am. J. Physiol.* **269** (1995) R630-R640.

[9]   H. Rupp, T.P. Rupp, B. Maisch. Fatty acid oxidation inhibition with PPARalpha activation (FOXIB/PPARalpha) for normalizing gene expression in heart failure? *Cardiovasc. Res.* **66** (2005) 423-426.

[10]   W. Grimm, M. Christ, J. Bach *et al.* Noninvasive arrhythmia risk stratification in idiopathic dilated cardiomyopathy: results of the Marburg Cardiomyopathy Study. *Circulation* **108** (2003) 2883-2891.

[11]   P.J. de Kam, G.L. Nicolosi, A.A. Voors *et al.* Prediction of 6 months left ventricular dilatation after myocardial infarction in relation to cardiac morbidity and mortality. Application of a new dilatation model to GISSI-3 data. *Eur. Heart J.* **23** (2002) 536-542.

[12]   P. Gaudron, I. Kugler, K. Hu *et al.* Time course of cardiac structural, functional and electrical changes in asymptomatic patients after myocardial infarction: their inter-relation and prognostic impact. *J. Am. Coll. Cardiol.* **38** (2001) 33-40.

[13]   M.R. Franz, R. Cima, D. Wang *et al.* Electrophysiological effects of myocardial stretch and mechanical determinants of stretch-activated arrhythmias. *Circulation* **86** (1992) 968-978.

[14]   Z. Wang, L.K. Taylor, W.D. Denney *et al.* Initiation of ventricular extrasystoles by myocardial stretch in chronically dilated and failing canine left ventricle. *Circulation* **90** (1994) 2022-2031.

[15]   M.F. Hazinski, A.H. Idris, R.E. Kerber *et al.* Lay rescuer automated external defibrillator ("public access defibrillation") programs: lessons learned from an international multicenter trial: advisory statement from the American Heart Association Emergency Cardiovascular Committee; the Council on Cardiopulmonary, Perioperative, and Critical Care; and the Council on Clinical Cardiology. *Circulation* **111** (2005) 3336-3340.

[16]   J.J. de Vreede-Swagemakers, A.P. Gorgels, W.I. Dubois-Arbouw *et al.* Out-of-hospital cardiac arrest in the 1990's: a population-based study in the Maastricht area on incidence, characteristics and survival. *J. Am. Coll. Cardiol.* **30** (1997) 1500-1505.

[17]   A. Dotevall, S. Johansson, L. Wilhelmsen *et al.* Increased levels of triglycerides, BMI and blood pressure and low physical activity increase the risk of diabetes in Swedish women. A prospective 18-year follow-up of the BEDA*study. *Diabet. Med.* **21** (2004) 615-622.

[18]   C.N. Verboom, R. Marchioli, H. Rupp *et al.* Highly purified omega-3 fatty acids for secondary prevention of post-myocardial infarction. Royal Society of Medicine Press, London (2003).

[19]   H. Rupp, C.N. Verboom, B. Jaeger. Saving lives post-MI: highly purified omega-3 PUFAs for the prevention of sudden death. *J. Clin. Basic Cardiol.* **5** (2002) 209-214.

[20]   GISSI-Prevenzione Investigators. Dietary supplementation with n-3 polyunsaturated fatty acids and vitamin E after myocardial infarction: results of the GISSI-Prevenzione trial. Gruppo Italiano per lo Studio della Sopravvivenza nell'Infarto miocardico. *Lancet* **354** (1999) 447-455.

[21]   J. Folch, M. Lees, G.H. Sloane Stanley. A simple method for the isolation and purification of total lipides from animal tissues. *J. Biol. Chem.* **226** (1957) 497-509.

[22]   W.K. Fulk and M.S. Shorb. Production of an artifact during methanolysis of lipids by boron trifluoride-methanol. *J. Lipid Res.* **11** (1970) 276-277.

[23]   C. Stavarache, M. Vinatoru, Y. Maeda. Ultrasonic versus silent methylation of vegetable oils. *Ultrason Sonochem* **13** (2006) 401-407.

[24]   H. Rupp, D. Wagner, T. Rupp *et al.* B. Risk stratification by the "EPA+DHA level" and the "EPA/AA ratio" focus on anti-inflammatory and antiarrhythmogenic effects of long-chain omega-3 fatty acids. *Herz* **29** (2004) 673-685.

[25]   C.M. Albert, H. Campos, M.J. Stampfer *et al.* Blood levels of long-chain n-3 fatty acids and the risk of sudden death. *N. Engl. J. Med.* **346** (2002) 1113-1118.

[26]   R. Marchioli, F. Avanzini, F. Barzi *et al.* Assessment of absolute risk of death after myocardial infarction by use of multiple-risk-factor assessment equations: GISSI-Prevenzione mortality risk chart. *Eur. Heart J.* **22** (2001) 2085-2103.

[27]   R. Marchioli, F. Barzi, E. Bomba *et al.* Early protection against sudden death by n-3 polyunsaturated fatty acids after myocardial infarction: time-course analysis of the results of the Gruppo Italiano per lo Studio della Sopravvivenza nell'Infarto Miocardico (GISSI)-Prevenzione. *Circulation* **105** (2002) 1897-1903.

[28]   D. Di Stasi, R. Bernasconi, R. Marchioli *et al.* Early modifications of fatty acid composition in plasma phospholipids, platelets and mononucleates of healthy volunteers after low doses of n-3 polyunsaturated fatty acids. *Eur. J. Clin. Pharmacol.* **60** (2004) 183-190.

[29]   D.S. Siscovick, T.E. Raghunathan, I. King *et al.* Dietary intake and cell membrane levels of long-chain n-3 polyunsaturated fatty acids and the risk of primary cardiac arrest. *JAMA* **274** (1995) 1363-1367.

[30]   D.W. Nilsen and W.S. Harris. n-3 Fatty acids and cardiovascular disease. *Am. J. Clin. Nutr.* **79** (2004) 166.

[31]   J.V. Donadio Jr, T.S. Larson, E.J. Bergstralh *et al.* A randomized trial of high-dose compared with low-dose omega-3 fatty acids in severe IgA nephropathy. *J. Am. Soc. Nephrol.* **12** (2001) 791-799.

[32]   E. Guallar, C.H. Hennekens, F.M. Sacks *et al.* A prospective study of plasma fish oil levels and incidence of myocardial infarction in U.S. male physicians. *J. Am. Coll. Cardiol.* **25** (1995) 387-394.

[33]   G.C. Leng, G.S. Taylor, A.J. Lee *et al.* Essential fatty acids and cardiovascular disease: the Edinburgh Artery Study. *Vasc. Med.* **4** (1999) 219-226.

[34]   P.J. Robinson, J. Noronha, J.J. DeGeorge *et al.* A quantitative method for measuring regional in vivo fatty-acid incorporation into and turnover within brain phospholipids: review and critical analysis. *Brain Res. Brain Res. Rev.* **17** (1992) 187-214.

[35]   S.S. Nair, J. Leitch, J. Falconer *et al.* Cardiac (n-3) non-esterified fatty acids are selectively increased in fish oil-fed pigs following myocardial ischemia. *J. Nutr.* **129** (1999) 1518-1523.

[36]   G.E. Billman, H. Hallaq, A. Leaf. Prevention of ischemia-induced ventricular fibrillation by omega 3 fatty acids. *Proc. Natl. Acad. Sci. U.S.A.* **91** (1994) 4427-4430.

[37]   R. Schrepf, T. Limmert, P. Claus Weber *et al.* Immediate effects of n-3 fatty acid infusion on the induction of sustained ventricular tachycardia. *Lancet* **363** (2004) 1441-1442.

[38]   A. Leaf, Y.F. Xiao, J.X. Kang *et al.* Prevention of sudden cardiac death by n-3 polyunsaturated fatty acids. *Pharmacol. Ther.* **98** (2003) 355-377.

[39]   H. Rupp, R. Wahl, M. Hansen. Influence of diet and carnitine palmitoyltransferase I inhibition on myosin and sarcoplasmic reticulum. *J. Appl. Physiol.* **72** (1992) 352-360.

[40]   D. von Au, M. Brändle, H. Rupp *et al.* Influence of a diet rich in fish oil on blood pressure, body weight and cardiac hypertrophy in spontaneously hypertensive rats. *Eur. J. Appl. Physiol. Occup. Physiol.* **58** (1988) 97-99.

[41]   R. Jacob, M. Brändle, B. Dierberger *et al.* Antihypertensive und kardioprotektive Effekte verschiedener Öldiäten. In: D. Ganten, G. Mall (Eds): *Herz-Kreislauf-Regulation, Organprotektion und Organschäden.* Schattauer Verlag, Stuttgart (1991) 25-46.

[42]   S. al Makdessi, M. Brändle, M. Ehrt *et al.* Myocardial protection by ischemic preconditioning: the influence of the composition of myocardial phospholipids. *Mol. Cell. Biochem.* **145** (1995) 69-73.

[43]   R. Eickhorn, H. Isensee, R. Jacob *et al.* No obvious influence of dietary fatty acid intake on cardiac sodium current of the rat. *Pflugers Arch.* **420 (suppl. 1)** (1992) 334.

[44]   Y.F. Xiao, J.X. Kang, J.P. Morgan *et al.* Blocking effects of polyunsaturated fatty acids on Na+ channels of neonatal rat ventricular myocytes. *Proc. Natl. Acad. Sci. U.S.A.* **92** (1995) 11000-11004.

[45]   Y.F. Xiao, Q. Ke, Y. Chen *et al.* Inhibitory effect of n-3 fish oil fatty acids on cardiac Na+/Ca2+ exchange currents in HEK293t cells. *Biochem. Biophys. Res. Commun.* **321** (2004) 116-123.

[46]   Y.F. Xiao, A.M. Gomez, J.P. Morgan *et al.* Suppression of voltage-gated L-type Ca2+ currents by polyunsaturated fatty acids in adult and neonatal rat ventricular myocytes. *Proc. Natl. Acad. Sci. U.S.A.* **94** (1997) 4182-4187.

[47]   K.Y. Bogdanov, H.A. Spurgeon, T.M. Vinogradova *et al.* Modulation of the transient outward current in adult rat ventricular myocytes by polyunsaturated fatty acids. *Am. J. Physiol.* **274** (1998) H571-H579.

[48]   E. Honore, J. Barhanin, B. Attali *et al.* External blockade of the major cardiac delayed-rectifier K+ channel (Kv1.5) by polyunsaturated fatty acids. *Proc. Natl. Acad. Sci. U.S.A.* **91** (1994) 1937-1941.

[49]   S.C. O'Neill, M.R. Perez, K.E. Hammond *et al.* Direct and indirect modulation of rat cardiac sarcoplasmic reticulum function by n-3 polyunsaturated fatty acids. *J. Physiol.* **538** (2002) 179-184.

[50]   J.S. Swan, K. Dibb, N. Negretti *et al.* Effects of eicosapentaenoic acid on cardiac SR Ca(2+)-release and ryanodine receptor function. *Cardiovasc. Res.* **60** (2003) 337-346.

[51]   M.H. Raitt, W.E. Connor, C. Morris *et al.* Fish oil supplementation and risk of ventricular tachycardia and ventricular fibrillation in patients with implantable defibrillators: a randomized controlled trial. *JAMA* **293** (2005) 2884-2891.

[52]   A. Leaf, C.M. Albert, M. Josephson *et al.* Prevention of fatal arrhythmias in high-risk subjects by fish oil n-3 fatty acid intake. *Circulation* **112** (2005) 2762-2768.

[53]   L. Calo, L. Bianconi, F. Colivicchi *et al.* N-3 fatty acids for the prevention of atrial fibrillation after coronary artery bypass surgery: a randomized, controlled trial. *J. Am. Coll. Cardiol.* **45** (2005) 1723-1728.

[54]   C. Pater, D. Compagnone, J. Luszick *et al.* Effect of Omacor on HRV parameters in patients with recent uncomplicated myocardial infarction - A randomized, parallel group, double-blind, placebo-controlled trial: study design [ISRCTN75358739]. *Curr. Control Trials Cardiovasc. Med.* **4** (2003) 2.

[55]   S. Pepe and P.L. McLennan. Cardiac membrane fatty acid composition modulates myocardial oxygen consumption and postischemic recovery of contractile function. *Circulation* **105** (2002) 2303-2308.

[56]   D. Rousseau, D. Moreau, D. Raederstorff *et al.* Is a dietary n-3 fatty acid supplement able to influence the cardiac effect of the psychological stress? *Mol. Cell. Biochem.* **178** (1998) 353-366.

[57]   M. Brändle and R. Jacob. Effects of a diet rich in Q-3 fatty acids on left ventricular geometry and dynamics in spontaneously hypertensive rats. *Eur. J. Appl. Physiol. Occup. Physiol.* **61** (1990) 177-181.

[58]   M. Kaieda, T. Samukawa, A. Kondo *et al.* Effect of methanol and water contents on production of biodiesel fuel from plant oil catalyzed by various lipases in a solvent-free system. *J. Biosci. Bioeng.* **91** (2001) 12-15.

[59]   L.D. Lawson and B.G. Hughes. Human absorption of fish oil fatty acids as triacylglycerols, free acids, or ethyl esters. *Biochem. Biophys. Res. Commun.* **152** (1988) 328-335.

[60]   L.D. Lawson and B.G. Hughes. Absorption of eicosapentaenoic acid and docosahexaenoic acid from fish oil triacylglycerols or fish oil ethyl esters co-ingested with a high-fat meal. *Biochem. Biophys. Res. Commun.* **156** (1988) 960-963.

[61]   S. el Boustani, C. Colette, L. Monnier *et al.* Enteral absorption in man of eicosapentaenoic acid in different chemical forms. *Lipids* **22** (1987) 711-714.

[62]   C. Luley, H. Wieland, J. Grünwald. Bioavailability of omega-3 fatty acids: ethylester preparations are as suitable as triglyceride preparations. *Akt. Ernähr-Med.* **15** (1990) 123-125.

[63]   I. Ikeda, Y. Imasato, H. Nagao *et al.* Lymphatic transport of eicosapentaenoic and docosahexaenoic acids as triglyceride, ethyl ester and free acid, and their effect on cholesterol transport in rats. *Life Sci.* **52** (1993) 1371-1379.

[64]   M. Kozak, L. Krivan, B. Semrad. Circadian variations in the occurrence of ventricular tachyarrhythmias in patients with implantable cardioverter defibrillators. *Pacing Clin. Electrophysiol.* **26** (2003) 731-735.

[65]   Die Nationale Verzehrsstudie. Bremerhaven: Wirtschaftsverlag NW (1991).

[66]   G.B. Mensink, M. Thamm, K. Haas. [Nutrition in Germany 1998]. *Gesundheitswesen* **61** (1999) S200-S206.

[67]   D. Kromhout, E.B. Bosschieter, C. de Lezenne Coulander. The inverse relation between fish consumption and 20-year mortality from coronary heart disease. *N. Engl. J. Med.* **312** (1985) 1205-1209.

[68]   D. Mozaffarian, R.N. Lemaitre, L.H. Kuller *et al.* Cardiac benefits of fish consumption may depend on the type of fish meal consumed: the Cardiovascular Health Study. *Circulation* **107** (2003) 1372-1377.

[69]   F.B. Hu, E. Cho, K.M. Rexrode *et al.* Fish and long-chain omega-3 fatty acid intake and risk of coronary heart disease and total mortality in diabetic women. *Circulation* **107** (2003) 1852-1857.

[70]   K. He, Y. Song, M.L. Daviglus *et al.* Accumulated evidence on fish consumption and coronary heart disease mortality: a meta-analysis of cohort studies. *Circulation* **109** (2004) 2705-2711.

[71]   C. von Schacky, P. Angerer, W. Kothny *et al.* The effect of dietary omega-3 fatty acids on coronary atherosclerosis. A randomized, double-blind, placebo-controlled trial. *Ann. Intern. Med.* **130** (1999) 554-562.

[72]   P.M. Kris-Etherton, W.S. Harris, L.J. Appel. Fish consumption, fish oil, omega-3 fatty acids, and cardiovascular disease. *Circulation* **106** (2002) 2747-2757.

[73]   F. van de Werf, D. Ardissino, A. Betriu *et al.* Management of acute myocardial infarction in patients presenting with ST-segment elevation. The Task Force on the Management of Acute Myocardial Infarction of the European Society of Cardiology. *Eur. Heart J.* **24** (2003) 28-66.

[74]   S. Yoon, A.E. Albers, A.P. Wong *et al.* Screening mercury levels in fish with a selective fluorescent chemosensor. *J. Am. Chem. Soc.* **127** (2005) 16030-16031.

[75]   J.M. Hightower and D. Moore. Mercury levels in high-end consumers of fish. *Environ. Health Perspect.* **111** (2003) 604-608.

[76]   J.F. Wilson. Balancing the risks and benefits of fish consumption. *Ann. Intern. Med.* **141** (2004) 977-980.

[77]   C. Despres, A. Beuter, F. Richer *et al.* Neuromotor functions in Inuit preschool children exposed to Pb, PCBs, and Hg. *Neurotoxicol. Teratol.* **27** (2005) 245-257.

[78]   E. Guallar, M.I. Sanz-Gallardo, P. van 't Veer *et al.* Mercury, fish oils, and the risk of myocardial infarction. *N. Engl. J. Med.* **347** (2002) 1747-1754.

[79]   J.T. Cohen, D.C. Bellinger, W.E. Connor *et al.* A quantitative risk-benefit analysis of changes in population fish consumption. *Am. J. Prev. Med.* **29** (2005) 325-334.

[80]   S.F. Melanson, E.L. Lewandrowski, J.G. Flood *et al.* Measurement of organochlorines in commercial over-the-counter fish oil preparations: implications for dietary and therapeutic recommendations for omega-3 fatty acids and a review of the literature. *Arch. Pathol. Lab. Med.* **129** (2005) 74-77.

[81]   H. Rupp, M. Turcani, T. Ohkubo *et al.* Dietary linolenic acid-mediated increase in vascular prostacyclin formation. *Mol. Cell. Biochem.* **162** (1996) 59-64.

[82]   E. Ros, I. Nunez, A. Perez-Heras *et al.* A walnut diet improves endothelial function in hypercholesterolemic subjects: a randomized crossover trial. *Circulation* **109** (2004) 1609-1614.

[83] H. Sprecher. An update on the pathways of polyunsaturated fatty acid metabolism. *Curr. Opin. Clin. Nutr. Metab. Care* **2** (1999) 135-138.

[84] R.K. Berge, L. Madsen, H. Vaagenes *et al.* In contrast with docosahexaenoic acid, eicosapentaenoic acid and hypolipidaemic derivatives decrease hepatic synthesis and secretion of triacylglycerol by decreased diacylglycerol acyltransferase activity and stimulation of fatty acid oxidation. *Biochem. J.* **343** (1999) 191-197.

[85] M.N. Sack, T.A. Rader, S. Park *et al.* Fatty acid oxidation enzyme gene expression is downregulated in the failing heart. *Circulation* **94** (1996) 2837-2842.

[86] H. Gerster. Can adults adequately convert alpha-linolenic acid (18:3n-3) to eicosapentaenoic acid (20:5n-3) and docosahexaenoic acid (22:6n-3)? *Int. J. Vitam. Nutr. Res.* **68** (1998) 159-173.

[87] G.C. Burdge and S.A. Wootton. Conversion of alpha-linolenic acid to eicosapentaenoic, docosapentaenoic and docosahexaenoic acids in young women. *Br. J. Nutr.* **88** (2002) 411-420.

[88] C. von Schacky and P.C. Weber. Metabolism and effects on platelet function of the purified eicosapentaenoic and docosahexaenoic acids in humans. *J. Clin. Invest.* **76** (1985) 2446-2450.

[89] M. Studer, M. Briel, B. Leimenstoll *et al.* Effect of different antilipidemic agents and diets on mortality: a systematic review. *Arch. Intern. Med.* **165** (2005) 725-730.

[90] W.S. Harris and C. von Schacky. The Omega-3 Index: a new risk factor for death from coronary heart disease? *Prev. Med.* **39** (2004) 212-220.

[91] D.W. Nilsen, G. Albrektsen, K. Landmark *et al.* Effects of a high-dose concentrate of n-3 fatty acids or corn oil introduced early after an acute myocardial infarction on serum triacylglycerol and HDL cholesterol. *Am. J. Clin. Nutr.* **74** (2001) 50-56.

[92] P. Yli-Jama, H.E. Meyer, J. Ringstad *et al.* Serum free fatty acid pattern and risk of myocardial infarction: a case-control study. *J. Intern. Med.* **251** (2002) 19-28.

[93] A. Macchia, G. Levantesi, M.G. Franzosi *et al.* Left ventricular systolic dysfunction, total mortality, and sudden death in patients with myocardial infarction treated with n-3 polyunsaturated fatty acids. *Eur. J. Heart Fail.* **7** (2005) 904-909.

Highly Purified Omega-3 Polyunsaturated Fatty Acids Are Effective as Adjunct Therapy for Secondary Prevention of Myocardial Infarction: Critical Analysis of GISSI-Prevenzione Trial

Cees N. Verboom
Solvay Pharmaceuticals, Hans-Böckler-Allee 20, 30173 Hannover, Germany

Abstract. Gruppo Italiano per lo Studio della Sopravvivenza nell'Infarto Miocardico (GISSI)-Prevenzione was the first large randomized trial to produce evidence that a pharmaceutical preparation of highly purified omega-3 polyunsaturated fatty acids (PUFAs), administered as an adjunct to other accepted interventions, had a favorable effect on hard clinical end-points in post-myocardial infarction patients. Much of the 20% all-cause mortality benefit recorded during the study could be attributed to a 45% reduction in sudden death - a fatal outcome that traditionally has proved resistant to medical intervention. These results were obtained with an omega-3 PUFA dose of 1 g/day, which is much lower than was routinely being used at the time the study was initiated (e.g. 4 g/day for hypertriglyceridemia). One consequence of this low-dose regimen was that the tolerability profile of omega-3 PUFAs during GISSI-Prevenzione was considered highly satisfactory, with low adverse event incidence rates and low rates of discontinuation due to adverse events. Time-course analysis established that much of the survival benefit of omega-3 PUFA treatment in GISSI-Prevenzione was realized during the early months of the trial. The beneficial effects of omega-3 PUFA treatment were observed on top of standard, secondary pharmacological prevention therapy like anti-platelet agents, statins, beta-blockers and angiotensin-converting enzyme (ACE) inhibitors. The benefits of omega-3 PUFA therapy were also apparent in patients at all standards of adherence to a healthy diet and may have been augmented in patients with the best dietary profile. Patients with diabetes mellitus ($\approx$15% of the study cohort) appeared to benefit from omega-3 PUFAs to at least the same extent as the general study population; the treatment effect on sudden death was progressively more pronounced as left ejection fraction declined. Cost-effectiveness analyses undertaken from a third-party payer perspective for Italy revealed that the cost of low-dose treatment with highly purified omega-3 PUFAs was approximately € 25,000 per life-year gained.

Keywords. GISSI-Prevenzione, highly purified omega-3 polyunsaturated fatty acids, randomized trial, all-cause mortality, sudden death, post-myocardial infarction, secondary prevention, diet, cost-effectiveness

1. GISSI-Prevenzione: Background and Guiding Principles of the Study

GISSI-Prevenzione was a multicenter study of the impact of highly purified omega-3 polyunsaturated fatty acids (PUFAs) on the prognosis of patients who had survived a recent myocardial infarction (MI), undertaken in the context of prevailing contemporary secondary preventive practice. The study was devised and conducted under the auspices of the Gruppo Italiano per lo Studio della Sopravvivenza nell'Infarto Miocardico (GISSI), itself the product of a collaboration between the Mario Negri Institute and the Associazione Nazionale dei Medici Cardiologi Ospedalieri (ANMCO) of Italy. Pragmatism and general applicability of findings are hallmarks of GISSI-sponsored studies [1-3] and GISSI-Prevenzione was no exception to these precepts. Accordingly, no age limits were specified and exclusion criteria were kept to a minimum: patients with a recent MI ($\leq$3 months) were eligible to participate in GISSI-Prevenzione provided they had no condition associated with poor short-term prognosis (including, but not limited to, congestive heart failure or cancer), no known contraindications to the study medications and no known congenital coagulation defect [4]. Use of drugs for secondary prevention (e.g. anti-platelet drugs, beta-blockers and angiotensin-converting enzyme (ACE) inhibitors) was permitted according to standard practice and at the discretion of individual investigators. As part of this optimized preventive regimen, patients were encouraged to adhere to a Mediterranean-style diet, with a high content of fruit, fish and fiber, and a relatively low content of saturated fats and red meat.

1.1. Summary of Study Design

GISSI-Prevenzione was conducted according to a PROBE (Prospective Randomized Open, with Blinded End-point adjudication) design in which treatments were administered open-label with ascertainment of prospectively defined end-points by a blinded End-point Validation Committee. A similar methodology has been successfully applied in other influential cardiovascular trials [e.g. 5]. A total of 11,323 patients were recruited and randomized at 172 participating clinical centers, making GISSI-Prevenzione one of the largest studies in secondary prevention. Randomization was preformed centrally, at the study co-ordinating center. Treatment assignment is summarized in Figure 1. Study medications comprised highly purified omega-3 PUFAs (84% eicosapentaenoic acid (EPA) and docosahexaenoic acid (DHA)), administered at a dose of 1 g/day, and vitamin E, administered as alpha-tocopherol (300 mg/day). In the Diet And Reinfarction Trial (DART) trial, a 29% reduction in 2 years all-cause mortality was seen in subjects advised to eat fatty fish compared with those not so advised [6]. The amount of fish in this study supplied 2.5 g EPA per week. One capsule highly purified omega-3 PUFAs given for seven days supplies approximately the same amount of EPA. At the start of the GISSI-P trial, controlled trials testing the effect of vitamin E on the incidence of cardiovascular events produced controversial effects. The combination arm was included, because a possible complimentary role of omega-3 PUFAs and vitamin E could not be excluded at the start of the trial. These interventions were added to prevailing standard medications for secondary prevention; the control group received conventional therapy only (Figure 1). None of the study groups received placebo. The number of patients lost to follow-up was remarkable low in the trial, only 13 of the 11,324 patients randomized.

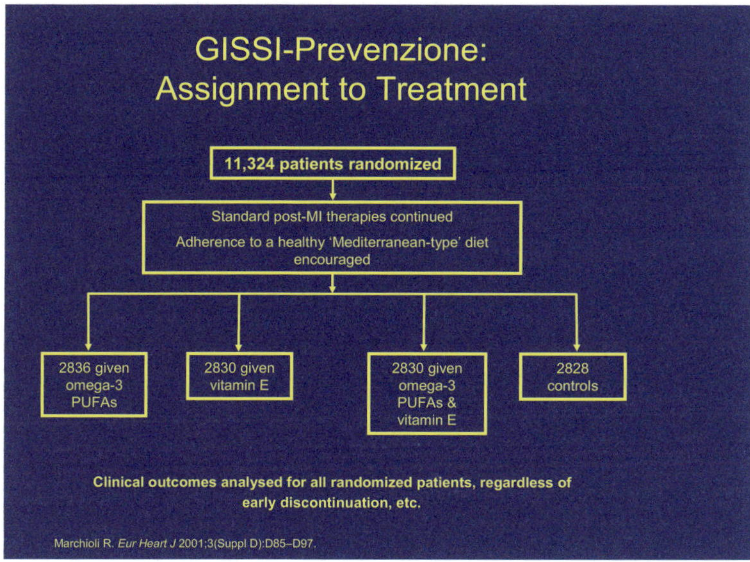

Figure 1. Summary of treatment assignments in GISSI-Prevenzione. PUFA = polyunsaturated fatty acid. Data from Ref. [4].

1.2. Patient Profile

Baseline characteristics of participating patients are shown in Tables 1 and 2 [4,7]. The patient population included in the trial can be characterized as relative low risk group, with 15% older than 70 years, 14% with echo-documented left ventricular ejection fraction of 40% or less, 29% with positive exercise tests and approximately 15% with diabetes mellitus as secondary diagnosis. 50% of the patients were recruited within 16 days after the myocardial infarction. Average baseline lipoprotein levels were higher than might be considered desirable for post-MI patients [8], but use of recommended preventive therapies at baseline was generally high, particularly in the case of anti-platelet agents. The emergence of lipid-lowering therapy as an accepted element of secondary prevention [9-13] was reflected in trend rates for the use of statins in the omega-3 PUFA cohort, which increased from less than 5% at the start of GISSI-Prevenzione to nearly 50% at completion of follow-up. This increasing use of statins during the trial is unlikely to have influenced the results of the study, as there was no substantial imbalance in their prescription between the different study groups.

Table 1. Baseline characteristics of patients in the GISSI-Prevenzione study. Data are given as means ± SD, where applicable. Data from Ref. [4,7]

	Omega-3 PUFAs (n = 2836)	Vitamin E (n = 2830)	PUFAs + vitamin E (n = 2830)	Conventional therapy (n = 2828)
No. males/females	2403/433	2398/432	2451/379	2407/421
Age (years)	59.4 ± 10.7	59.5 ± 10.5	59.1 ± 10.4	59.4 ± 10.5
Days since diagnosis of index MI	25.4 ± 21.0	25.0 ± 20.7	24.7 ± 20.7	25.2 ± 21.2
Body-mass index (kg/m^2)	26.5 ± 3.9	26.5 ± 3.6	26.6 ± 3.6	26.4 ± 3.5
Body-mass index >30 kg/m^2; n (%)	419 (14.9)	403 (14.4)	432 (15.5)	390 (14.0)
Ejection fraction	52.6 ± 10.6	52.9 ± 10.5	52.4 ± 10.4	52.5 ± 10.8
Ejection fraction <40%; n (%)	339 (14%)	314 (13.1%)	338 (14.1)	329 (13.7)
Total cholesterol (mg/dl)	210.2 ± 42.2	211.0 ± 42.4	210.6 ± 41.5	211.6 ± 42.3
LDL cholesterol (mg/dl)	136.3 ± 38.7	137.4 ± 38.0	137.6 ± 37.9	138.1 ± 37.5
HDL cholesterol (mg/dl)	41.5 ± 11.3	41.3 ± 11.2	41.6 ± 11.5	41.7 ± 12.0
Triglycerides (mg/dl)	162.6 ± 81.7	163.3 ± 85.3	160.3 ± 80.3	161.9 ± 94.4
Secondary diagnoses; n (%)				
Hypertension	1019 (35.9)	1007 (35.6)	1033 (36.5)	967 (34.2)
Diabetes mellitus	405 (14.3)	426 (15.1)	426 (15.1)	426 (15.1)
Smokers	1190 (42.3)	1161 (41.3)	1233 (43.5)	1234 (44.0)
Non-smokers	632 (22.4)	636 (22.6)	618 (22.0)	613 (21.9)
Ex-smokers	994 (35.3)	1016 (36.1)	972 (34.5)	953 (34.0)
>10 PVC/hour	259 (13.1)	252 (12.6)	278 (14.1)	279 (14.1)
Positive exercise-stress test	550 (29.8)	511 (27.8)	542 (29.0)	543 (29.0)

LDL = low-density lipoprotein; HDL = high-density lipoprotein; MI = myocardial infarction; PUFA = polyunsaturated fatty acid; PVC = premature ventricular contractions.

Table 2. Summary of usage of secondary preventive medication at baseline and during the GISSI-Prevenzione study. Data from Ref. [4,7]

	Omega-3 PUFAs (n = 2835)	Vitamin E (n = 2830)	PUFAs + vitamin E (n = 2830)	Conventional therapy (n = 2828)
Anti-platelet agents; n (%)				
Baseline	2600 (91.7)	2565 (90.6)	2582 (91.2)	2562 (90.6)
6 months	2309 (88.2)	2262 (87.4)	2260 (87.5)	2267 (88.3)
42 months	1714 (83.4)	1660 (82.7)	1691 (83.2)	1634 (82.1)
ACE-inhibitors; n (%)				
Baseline	1298 (46.0)	1287 (45.7)	1352 (48.1)	1343 (48.0)
6 months	1033 (39.4)	1074 (41.5)	1045 (40.4)	1083 (42.2)
42 months	791 (38.5)	783 (39.0)	829 (40.8)	759 (38.1)
Beta-blockers; n (%)				
Baseline	1237 (43.9)	1261 (44.8)	1250 (44.4)	1238 (44.2)
6 months	1092 (41.7)	1085 (41.9)	1052 (40.7)	1043 (40.6)
42 months	811 (39.5)	792 (39.4)	766 (37.7)	739 (37.1)
Cholesterol-lowering drugs; n (%)				
Baseline	124 (4.4)	130 (4.6)	135 (4.8)	145 (5.1)
6 months	784 (28.6)	781 (28.8)	758 (28.0)	786 (29.2)
42 months	1006 (46.0)	967 (44.9)	1017 (46.7)	944 (44.4)

ACE = angiotensin-converting enzyme; PUFA = polyunsaturated fatty acid.

Adherence to the advised diet, as represented by patient-reported consumption of sentinel foodstuffs, was high throughout the study and tended to improve with duration of follow-up [4,7]. (Data from exploratory analyses of the interaction between dietary status and clinical effects are discussed later in this chapter.)

2. GISSI-Prevenzione: Study End-Points

GISSI-Prevenzione had two pre-specified primary efficacy end-points:
1. Cumulative rate of all-cause mortality, non-fatal MI and non-fatal stroke.
2. Cumulative rate of cardiovascular mortality, non-fatal MI and non-fatal stroke.

Fatal cardiovascular end-point definitions were based on a nested classification (Figure 2) and identified via death certificates or hospital records. A non-fatal MI was diagnosed when a patient exhibited two or more of the following features:
- pathognomonic chest pain
- ST changes of 1 mm or more in any limb lead; or of more than 2 mm in any precordial lead; or both
- doubling or greater in diagnostic enzymes.

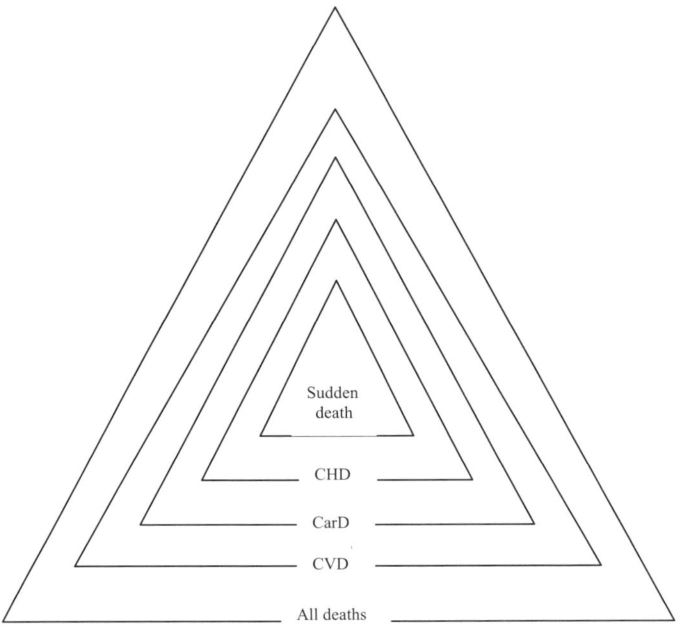

Figure 2. Inter-relationships of fatal end-points in the GISSI-Prevenzione study. All end-points were confirmed by a blinded End-point Validation Committee. CVD = cardiovascular (CV) death (any CV cause); CarD = cardiac death (any cardiac cause); CHD = coronary death (any coronary cause).

A non-fatal stroke was diagnosed if a patient exhibited unequivocal signs or symptoms of persisting neurological deficit with a sudden onset and a duration of at least 24 hours. A stroke was classified as fatal if a death certificate or relevant hospital records supplemented these diagnostic requirements. Secondary efficacy analyses included inspection of all components of the primary end-points and the principal causes of death.

2.1. GISSI-Prevenzione: Statistical Considerations and Methods

Statistical calculations were based on the assumption of a 20% cumulative event rate for the end-points of all-cause mortality plus non-fatal MI and non-fatal stroke in the control group during the anticipated follow-up interval of 42 months [4]. Accordingly the recruitment of approximately 3000 patients per group would endow the study with (a) sufficient statistical power to discern a 20% relative risk reduction for the combined primary end-point of all-cause mortality plus non-fatal MI and non-fatal stroke in any of the three treatment groups compared with the control group, and (b) sufficient statistical power to discern a 20% relative risk reduction for that primary end-point with combined therapy versus either monotherapy. Statistical comparisons emphasized four-way analysis, in which any treatment assignment could be compared with any other. Outcomes were analyzed according to the principles of intention-to-treat. Follow-up data were right-censored at 42 months, at which time vital status data were available for 99.9% of patients. More than 38,000 patient-years of data were accrued during an average 3.5 years of follow-up.

A series of exploratory analyses were also undertaken. The findings of these exercises are discussed later in this chapter.

3. Primary Results of GISSI-Prevenzione

3.1. Effects of Highly Purified Omega-3 PUFAs

Omega-3 PUFAs significantly reduced the risk of experiencing a primary end-point event in GISSI-Prevenzione. Compared with controls, the risk reduction for the end-point of all-cause mortality plus non-fatal MI and non-fatal stroke was 15% (p=0.023); the risk reduction for the other primary end-point of cardiovascular death plus non-fatal MI and non-fatal stroke was 20% (p=0.008) [4]. Further analysis revealed that the reduction in risk of primary end-point events by highly purified omega-3 PUFAs was due to a reduction in all-cause mortality (20% risk reduction; p=0.01) and in several categories of cardiovascular death, notably sudden death (45% risk reduction; p=0.010) [4]. There was no significant impact on patients' risk of experiencing a fatal or non-fatal stroke (Table 3). No significant difference was also observed in the patients undergoing percutaneous transluminal coronary angioplasty or coronary artery bypass graft, 588 patients (20.7%) in the omega-3 PUFAs group versus 575 (20.3%) in the control group (RR: 1.01 (0.90-1.14)) [7]. In contrast to the GISSI-Prevenzione study, Nilsen *et al* did not observe a clinical benefit of omega-3 fatty acids in post-MI patients [14]. In this study, patients with acute MI were randomized to a daily dose of 4 grams omega-3 fatty acids or placebo over 12-24 months. The study was performed in one center in Norway. An interesting hypothesis to explain the lack of beneficial effects was formulated by the investigators of the Nilsen study. In a retrospective analysis, they reported that in their study the EPA+DHA concentrations at baseline were approximately twice the concentrations reported in other studies, probably due to the high intake of fish by their patients who were recruited in Stavanger, Norway. The investigators postulated that there may be an upper limit of tissue omega-3 fatty acid concentrations above which further benefit will not be realized [15].

Table 3. Summary of primary and secondary end-point results in GISSI-Prevenzione. Data are derived from four-way analysis. Patients with two or more events of different types appear more than once in columns but once only in rows. Data from Ref. [4]

	Omega-3 PUFAs (n = 2836)	Conventional therapy (n = 2828)	Relative risk reduction[a] (95% CI)
Primary end-points; n (%)			
All-cause mortality, non-fatal MI and stroke	356 (12.3%)	414 (14.6%)	0.85 (0.74-0.98)
Cardiovascular mortality, non-fatal MI and stroke	262 (9.2%)	322 (11.4%)	0.80 (0.68-0.95)
Secondary end-points; n (%)			
All deaths	236 (8.3%)	293 (10.4%)	0.80 (0.67-0.94)
CVD death	136 (4.8%)	193 (6.8%)	0.70 (0.56-0.87)
Cardiac death	108 (3.8%)	165 (5.8%)	0.65 (0.51-0.82)
Coronary death	100 (3.5%)	151 (5.3%)	0.65 (0.51-0.84)
Sudden death	55 (1.9%)	99 (3.5%)	0.55 (0.40-0.76)
Non-fatal cardiovascular events	140 (4.9%)	144 (5.1%)	0.96 (0.76-1.21)
Death from other causes	100 (3.5%)	100 (3.5%)	0.99 (0.74-1.30)
Other analyses; n (%)			
CVD death & non-fatal MI	196 (6.9%)	259 (9.2%)	0.75 (0.62-0.90)
Fatal & non-fatal stroke	54 (1.9%)	41 (1.5%)	1.30 (0.87-1967)

[a]Ratio <1 favors omega-3 PUFAs.
CVD = cardiovascular disease; MI = myocardial infarction; PUFA = polyunsaturated fatty acid

3.2. Lipoprotein and Biochemistry Effects

Comparison of cholesterol data (total, HDL, and LDL) at baseline and after 6 months of treatment revealed no substantial effects of highly purified omega-3 PUFAs on these parameters at the dose administered in the trial. Control-adjusted levels of cholesterol lipoproteins did not change by more than 2.5%. Median triglyceride levels were reduced by less than 5% relative to the control group after 6 months of treatment [4]. Lipid trends during the whole study period are depicted in Figure 3 [16]. Total cholesterol and LDL cholesterol returned to approximately baseline levels, while HDL cholesterol increased in a similar way in the omega-3 PUFA-groups and the control group. There was a decrease in triglycerides of 4.6% in the omega-3 PUFA-group after 42 months, which was statistically but probably not clinically significant. Approximately 15% of the patients on omega-3 PUFA did have diabetes mellitus as a secondary diagnosis, however blood glucose levels and fibrinogen concentrations were not altered substantively during therapy. Also in the Diet And Reinfarction Trial the reduction in mortality was observed in the absence of a reduction in cholesterol [6].

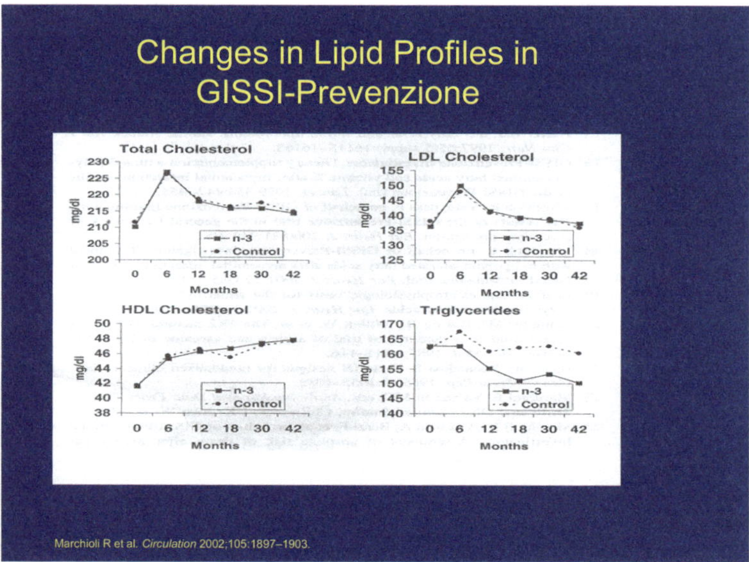

Figure 3. Trends in total and lipoprotein cholesterol and triglycerides during the GISSI-Prevenzione study. Control = patients who received standard post-myocardial infarction medications but neither highly purified omega-3 polyunsaturated fatty acids (PUFAs) nor vitamin E. Data from Ref. [16].

3.3. Tolerability and Safety

Highly purified omega-3 PUFAs were very well-tolerated during GISSI-Prevenzione. Gastrointestinal disturbances and nausea were the most frequent reported adverse events during the study, and the rate of discontinuation for treatment-related adverse events was very low (Table 4) [4]. Numbers of deaths due to non-cardiovascular causes were similar in both the omega-3 PUFA-group and the control group. This category of events therefore made no contribution to the superiority of highly purified omega-3 PUFAs over controls for the primary end-points of GISSI-Prevenzione. Cancer occurred in 61 (2.2%) patients in the control group and in 77 (2.7%) patients in the omega-3 PUFA-group. These data provided further reassurance, however, that there were no substantive non-cardiovascular safety concerns for the long-term use of highly purified omega-3 PUFAs. The rates of discontinuation for highly purified omega-3 PUFAs alone and vitamin E alone were, respectively, 11.6% and 7.3% after 1 year, and 28.5% and 26.2% over the entire course of the study [4].

Table 4. Highly purified omega-3 polyunsaturated fatty acids were well-tolerated in GISSI-Prevenzione, with a low rate of reported adverse events. Data from Ref. [4]

	Incidence (%)
Principal adverse events	
Gastrointestinal disturbances	4.9
Nausea	1.4
Discontinuation due to adverse events	3.8
Cumulative discontinuation from therapy after 3.5 years	28.5

3.4. Effects of Vitamin E or Combination Therapy

Vitamin E had no significant effect on either of the primary end-points of GISSI-Prevenzione and, unlike highly purified omega-3 PUFAs, no significant impact on all-cause mortality. Taken in conjunction with data from other, more recent, trials such as HOPE (Heart Outcomes Prevention Evaluation), the Heart Protection Study and the Women's Health Study [17-20], the results of GISSI-Prevenzione provide little reason to expect mortality benefits from vitamin E for the generality of patients with cardiovascular disease. Data from small trials in specific populations (e.g. patients undergoing hemodialysis [21]) keep open for the moment, however, the possibility that some specialist niches may exist for vitamin E in cardiovascular medicine. Combined therapy with highly purified omega-3 PUFAs plus vitamin E had effects similar to those of omega-3 PUFAs alone. There was no indication of any clinical synergism between the two treatments [4,7].

4. Exploratory Analyses

GISSI-Prevenzione is no exception to the principle that retrospective subgroup analyses lack statistical power and should not be regarded as definitive evidence for the existence or absence of a particular effect. Certain subsidiary analyses of the GISSI-database may nevertheless be informative to physicians seeking to assimilate the results of this study into their standard of care for post-MI patients.

4.1. Time-Course of Mortality Reduction

The observation that risk of a primary end-point event was reduced within a few months of starting highly purified omega-3 PUFA therapy stimulated a further analysis of factors contributing to this result [16]. A re-evaluation of all fatal outcomes was therefore undertaken, blinded to treatment assignment but with the aid of event data that became available after the completion of the primary analysis. Early trends in the various forms of cardiovascular mortality were examined in detail by right-censoring survival data at monthly intervals, beginning at the first month after randomization. This analysis confirmed an early treatment benefit on total survival that was both large and statistically significantly after 3 months (41% risk reduction vs. control group; p=0.037) and thereafter remained statistically significant and clinically meaningful for the remainder of the study (Figure 4a) [16]. The re-evaluation procedure described also confirmed 265 cases of sudden death during the study. A similar censored analysis of these events revealed an early effect of highly purified omega-3 PUFAs in reducing risk of sudden death, with a large and statistically significant benefit (53% risk reduction vs. controls; p=0.048) being apparent after 4 months (Figure 4b) [16]. The reduction in sudden death at 3 months, although narrowly failing the test of statistical significance (p=0.058), explained more than half of the reduction in total mortality at that time. By the end of follow-up at 42 months, the reduction in sudden death was highly statistically significant (p=0.0006) and accounted for 59% of the total survival benefit of highly purified omega-3 PUFAs seen during GISSI-Prevenzione. These data were interpreted by the investigators as evidence that much of the benefit of highly purified omega-3 PUFAs seen in GISSI-Prevenzione was attributable to an early and then sustained effect reducing the risk of sudden death. Lipid trends, already discussed in this chapter, and time trends for mortality benefit in patients randomized to omega-3 PUFA therapy in GISSI-Prevenzione, are not compatible with the accepted mode of benefit of statins. The results of a meta-analysis published in 2005 appear to support this view [22]. Researchers reported that omega-3 PUFAs reduced overall mortality risk by 23%, more than any of five other lipid-lowering interventions studied - but had almost no effect on plasma cholesterol levels (2% reduction) [22]. The pronounced impact of omega-3 PUFAs on mortality, despite little change in cholesterol, is markedly at variance with experience of statins where clinical benefit is closely linked to reductions in total and low-density lipoprotein cholesterol and beneficial occur after 1-2 years after the start of the treatment. A range of theories have been propounded to explain such an effect. Many of these emphasize the stabilization of electrically dysfunctional cardiomyocytes [23-28]. The fast effect of omega-3 PUFAs is in agreement with the effect seen in the Diet And Reinfarction Trial, in which the effect of fish advice on survival also appeared early and persisted up to 2 years [6].

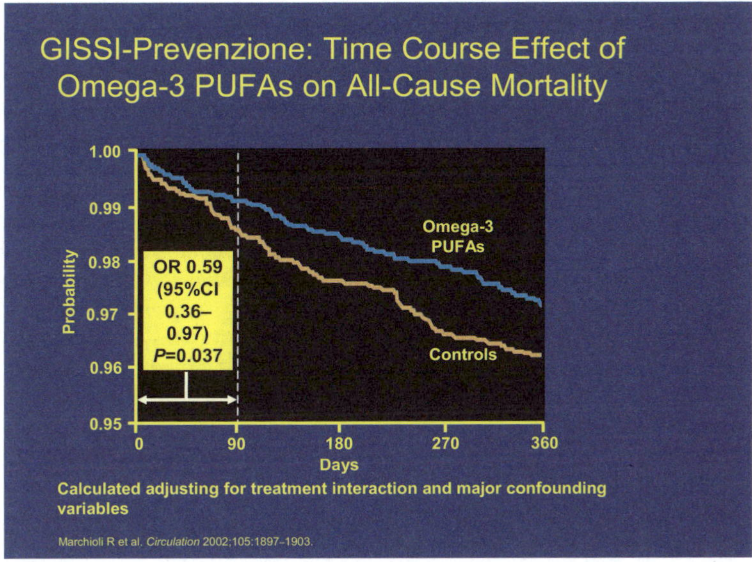

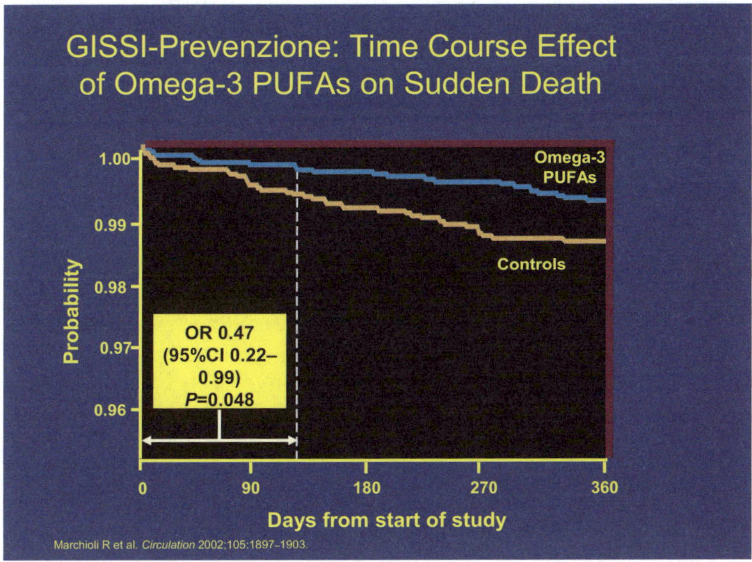

Figure 4. There was evidence for a significant reduction in total mortality with highly purified omega-3 polyunsaturated fatty acids (PUFAs) in the GISSI-Prevenzione study after 3 months of treatment (a), and evidence of a significant reduction in sudden death (b) after 4 months. Most of the early reduction in total mortality was attributable to a reduction in sudden death. Data from Ref. [16].

4.2. Outcomes in Patients with Low Baseline Ejection Fraction

The importance of left ventricular systolic dysfunction (defined as ejection fraction (EF) $\leq$40%, plus other functional indices) as a determinant of prognosis post-MI was re-affirmed during the development of a prediction model based on GISSI-Prevenzione data [29].

Subsequently, investigators examined the effects of highly purified omega-3 PUFA therapy on all-cause mortality and sudden death in patients stratified according to echocardiographically determined baseline left ventricular EF [30]. Using this criterion (and excluding patients for whom dyspnea data were not available (n = 9)), data were accrued from 9630 patients in the GISSI-Prevenzione population, representing 86% of the total study cohort. Inspection of patients stratified according to EF less than or greater than 50% revealed substantial statistical heterogeneity between the two patient subsets for an extensive range of clinical parameters, notably history of multiple MI or use of ACE-inhibitors (more prevalent in patients with ventricular dysfunction) and beta-blockers (less prevalent in patients with ventricular dysfunction). This imbalance was also evident for the end-points of all-cause mortality and sudden death, both of which occurred twice as frequently among patients with systolic ventricular dysfunction (p<0.0001 vs. patients with normal ventricular function). A series of Cox multivariable regression models correcting for these imbalances was used to investigate the relation between outcome and EF. Variables examined comprised:

- age and sex;
- the specific post-MI complications of: electrical instability, defined as 10 or more premature ventricular beats/hour or sustained repetitive arrhythmias during 24-hour monitoring; or residual ischemia according to specified criteria;
- the cardiovascular risk factors of smoking, history of diabetes or hypertension, total and high-density lipoprotein cholesterol, and presence of peripheral vascular disease;
- the treatment variables of anti-platelet drugs, beta-blockers and ACE-inhibitors.

After adjustment for these variables, left ventricular systolic dysfunction, as represented by EF, emerged as an independent predictor of both total mortality and sudden death, with the hazard ratio for both outcomes among patients with EF 35% or less being more than three times that in patients with EF greater than 50% [30]. In this situation, omega-3 PUFA therapy was associated with a reduction in overall mortality at all levels of ventricular function (test for heterogeneity >0.5). In respect of sudden death, however, there was a marked difference in treatment effect according to EF status: the relative risk reduction for sudden death among patients with EF less than 50% was 58% (p=0.0003), whereas among patients with well-preserved EF the relative risk reduction was 11% (p=0.071; test for heterogeneity 0.07). A synopsis of these data appears in Figures 5 & 6, which illustrate the fourfold greater reductions in relative risk of sudden death (Figure 5) and total mortality (Figure 6) in patients with low EF (≤40%) compared with those whose baseline EF was greater than 50%. These data were interpreted by GISSI-Prevenzione investigators as confirmation that the total mortality benefit of highly purified omega-3 PUFAs is conferred on patients with all grades of systolic ventricular function but that the benefit in terms of reduced risk of sudden death is sharply focused towards patients with impaired systolic function. Suggestions advanced to explain this duality of effect include the proposition that augmentation of cardiac electrical stability may dominate in patients with diminished EF (hence the greater effect on sudden death), whereas the reduction in all-cause mortality in patients with better-preserved ventricular function may arise from anti-inflammatory and plaque-stabilizing effects of omega-3 PUFAs [31-33], perhaps including contributions from the recently identified PUFA metabolites known as *resolvins* [34]. Further insights into the benefits and possible mechanisms of benefit of omega-3 PUFA therapy in patients with reduced left ventricular EF may emerge from the GISSI-HF study. This factorial, end-point-driven study with a planned duration of 3 years has been designed to investigate the effect of highly purified omega-3 PUFAs on total mortality and hospitalizations for cardiovascular reasons in approximately 7000 patients with a clinical diagnosis of heart failure. The impact of the lipid-lowering agent rosuvastatin on prognosis in heart failure will also be studied.

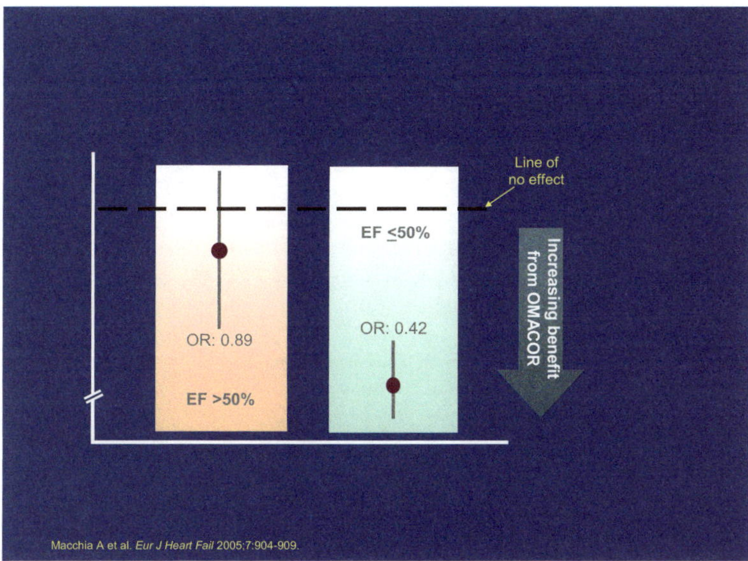

Figure 5. The treatment effect of highly purified omega-3 polyunsaturated fatty acids (PUFAs) on sudden death in GISSI-Prevenzione was greater in patients with low left ventricular ejection fraction (EF) than in patients with EF >50%. OR = odds ratio. Data from Ref. [30].

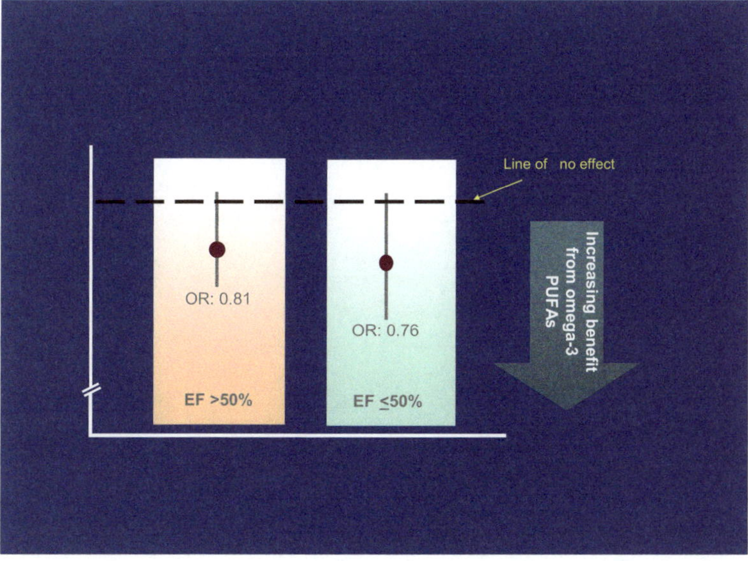

Figure 6. The treatment effect of highly purified omega-3 polyunsaturated fatty acids (PUFAs) on total mortality in GISSI-Prevenzione was greater in patients with low left ventricular ejection fraction (EF) than in patients with EF >50%. OR = odds ratio. Data from Ref. [30].

4.3. Interactions between Highly Purified Omega-3 PUFAs and Food

The influence of food habits on the clinical findings of the GISSI-Prevenzione study has been the subject of extended analysis. Barzi and colleagues [35] examined the relation between adherence to/compliance with a Mediterranean-type diet and all-cause mortality in the GISSI-Prevenzione population and reported that a greater observance of the principles of healthy eating was associated with a clear and progressive improvement in prognosis. The impact of the five sentinel foodstuffs used to monitor dietary practices is summarized in Table 5. As shown in the Table there was a compelling trend toward improved survival with a greater consumption of each category of foodstuff considered indicative of adherence to a healthy diet. Moreover, this trend was robust when adjusted for the potential confounding influence of a wide range of dietary and non-dietary factors (specified in Table 5). A plot of adjusted odds ratios (on a log-scale) versus dietary score confirmed a strong and consistent linear trend for better prognosis with better dietary habits.

Table 5. Relation between time-weighted average consumption of five sentinel foodstuffs and total mortality during the GISSI-Prevenzione study. Odds ratios shown are adjusted for: age, sex, history of hypertension or diabetes mellitus, smoking status, claudication, cardiac electrical instability, left ventricular dysfunction, residual myocardial ischemia, concomitant secondary preventive therapies, GISSI-Prevenzione study medication assignment, and the four other categories of examined foodstuffs. Data from Ref. [35]

	Adjusted odds ratio*			Adjusted odds ratio*
Fish			**Cooked vegetables**	
Never/seldom	1		Never/seldom	1
1 meal/week	0.83		2-3 portions/week	0.79
2 meals/week	0.73		1 portion/day	0.69
>2 meals/week	0.66		>1 portion/day	0.55
	P for trend <0.001			P for trend <0.0001
Fruit			**Raw vegetables**	
Never/seldom	1		Never/seldom	1
2-3 portions/week	0.80		2-3 portions/week	0.77
1 portion/day	0.75		1 portion/day	0.60
>1 portion/day	0.58		>1 portion/day	0.54
	P for trend <0.0001			P for trend <0.0001
Olive oil				
Never/seldom	1			
Often	0.77			
Regularly	0.71			
	P for trend <0.002			

*relative to 'never/seldom' category

These findings are consistent with an extensive literature that affirms the benefits of healthy eating for cardiac patients [6,36-39]. However, GISSI-Prevenzione enlarges on experience with dietary modification in several noteworthy ways. First, the substantial treatment benefit from omega-3 PUFAs in a population characterized by widespread use of a Mediterranean-type diet at baseline (and with further improvement in dietary profile during the study) indicates that low-dose omega-3 PUFAs confer greater survival benefits than are provided by dietary means alone, and highlights the desirability of including pharmaceutical omega-3 PUFA supplementation in standard medical regimens for secondary prevention. In addition, analysis of the impact of omega-3 PUFAs in patients stratified by quartiles of dietary adherence indicates that the benefits of low-dose omega-3 PUFA supplements are realized in patients with poor dietary profiles and may even be accentuated in those with the best dietary habits. The pragmatic interpretation of these findings is that use of supplementary omega-3 PUFAs is appropriate irrespective of dietary profile. From this it may be deduced that attainment of a good diet is not a reason to stop using low-dose omega-3 PUFAs. In fact, the prospect of additional benefit from low-dose omega-3 PUFA therapy might be used as an incentive to persist with good dietary habits.

4.4. Metabolic Syndrome and Risk of Cardiovascular Events after Myocardial Infarctions

In a retrospective, the investigators analyzed the prevalence and prognostic role of the metabolic syndrome (METS) and diabetes mellitus in the post-myocardial infarction patients enrolled in the GISSI-Prevenzione trial [40]. In the trial, insulin resistance was a common finding. At baseline, 2,139 (20.6%) and 3,047 (29.3%) of the patients had diabetes mellitus and METS respectively. As compared with METS and control subjects, diabetic patients were more likely to be female, older, and with higher prevalence of peripheral artery disease and myocardial infarction before the event leading to recruitment in the study. Diabetic patients were also more likely to have an impaired left ventricular function with lower levels of ejection fraction and higher prevalence of NYHA functional class II. The mean ejection fraction in diabetic patients was 51+/-11, versus 53+/-10 in the control group and in the METS patients (p=<0.00012). In comparison with control patients, the probability of death and a major cardiovascular events were higher in both the METS patients (+29%, p=0.002; +23%, p=0.005) and diabetic patients (+68%, p<0.0001; +47%, p<0.0001). Diabetic but not METS patients were more likely to be hospitalized for congestive heart failure (+89%, p=0.0003) and METS patients (+24%, p=0.241), as compared with controls. In addition METS patients had a near twofold increased risk of developing diabetes (+93%, p<0.0001). These results once again demonstrate that diabetes mellitus and METS are well-recognized risk factors for cardiovascular morbidity and mortality in patients who survived a myocardial infarction.

5. Cost-Effectiveness of Low-Dose Highly Purified Omega-3 PUFAs in Cardiovascular Secondary Prevention

Assessment of the cost-effectiveness of medications is now an integral element in the development of therapies in many industrialized nations. An appraisal of the cost-effectiveness of highly purified omega-3 PUFAs as an adjunct to standard secondary preventive measures post-MI has been undertaken based on data drawn directly from GISSI-Prevenzione [41]. Direct costs of hospital admissions, laboratory and diagnostic tests and other secondary preventive medications were acquired by taking usage data directly from GISSI-Prevenzione and applying costs based on diagnosis-related groups (for admissions and tests) or by applying the costs of defined daily dosages (for medications). Effectiveness was represented by the increase in life expectancy conferred by highly purified omega-3 PUFA therapy per patient over the course of the study (i.e. 3.5 years). The entire appraisal was undertaken from a third-party payer perspective using 1999 costs re-stated in Euros and discounted at 5% per annum. There were no significant differences between the highly purified omega-3 PUFA-treated patients and patients in the control group in respect of: number or frequency of hospital admissions for non-fatal events; proportion of patients using specified types of other preventive medications or duration of time for which those medications were prescribed; or costs due to laboratory or diagnostic tests. The difference in total per-capita cost of treatment between the highly purified omega-3 PUFA-treated and control patients (€ 817) was thus almost entirely due to the cost of highly purified omega-3 PUFAs (€ 803/year). Highly purified omega-3 PUFAs were calculated to confer an increment in life expectancy of 0.0332 years during 3.5 years of follow-up. The base-case cost per life-year gained was therefore € 24,603. Sensitivity analyses identified a cost per life-year gained ranging from € 15,721 to € 52,524 (Table 6). In an accompanying comparative analysis, the authors of this research calculated that 172 patients would have to be treated with highly purified omega-3 PUFAs for 1 year to save one patient. This number compared with 168 patients with simvastatin in the Scandinavian Simvastatin Survival Study (4S) trial [9], 202 treated with pravastatin in the Long-Term Prevention with Pravastatin in Ischaemic Disease (LIPID) trial [12] and 661 treated with pravastatin in the Cholesterol and Recurrent Events (CARE) trial [11]. The corresponding costs to save one patient were € 67,776 for highly purified omega-3 PUFAs, € 77,980 for simvastatin and € 189,879 and € 597,176 for pravastatin in LIPID and CARE, respectively [41].

Table 6. Highly purified omega-3 PUFA therapy for secondary prevention post-myocardial infarction (daily dose 1 g) was shown to be a cost-effective intervention in an analysis based on data derived from GISSI-Prevenzione. The most favorable outcome in sensitivity analysis was based on the best plausible estimate of clinical effectiveness and the lowest plausible estimate of costs, from the 4-way analysis; the least favorable outcome in sensitivity analysis was based on the worst plausible estimate of clinical effectiveness and the highest plausible estimate of costs, from the 2-way analysis. All costs and benefits were accrued over 3.5 years; base-case was discounted at 5% per annum. Data from Ref. [41]

	Incremental cost per patient (€)	Incremental effectiveness (life-years per patient)	Cost per life-year saved (€)
Base-case	817	0.0332	24,609
Best case	623	0.0396	15,721
Worst case	1129	0.0215	52,524

6. Conclusion

The results of the GISSI-Prevenzione study confirmed in a clinical setting a large repertoire of experimental evidence linking omega-3 PUFAs to improved cardiovascular prognosis and introduced omega-3 PUFA therapy as an important new and additional principle in secondary prevention post-MI. The fact that the improvement in overall survival was attributable to a significant and relatively early reduction in risk of sudden death - a form of death that has in the past proved particularly resistant to medical therapies - suggests a unique therapeutic niche for highly purified omega-3 PUFAs in the management of post-MI patients. It should be recalled that these effects were achieved in a patient population extensively medicated with other established drug therapies: it may be deduced from this that highly purified omega-3 PUFAs have effects additional to standard preventive therapies and should be considered as an adjunct to those treatments.

The case for using highly purified omega-3 PUFAs post-MI is further enhanced by the evidence from GISSI-Prevenzione that these agents are impressively well-tolerated when administered at a dose of 1 g/day and by the demonstration that highly purified omega-3 PUFAs satisfy current criteria for cost-effectiveness.

References

[1]   Gruppo Italiano per lo Studio della Streptochi-nasi nell'Infarto Miocardico (GISSI). Long-term effects of intravenous thrombolysis in acute myocardial infarction: final report of the GISSI study. *Lancet* **2** (1987) 871-874.

[2]   Gruppo Italiano per lo Studio della Sopravvivenza nell'Infarto Miocardico. GISSI-2: a factorial randomised trial of alteplase versus streptokinase and heparin versus no heparin among 12,490 patients with acute myocardial infarction. *Lancet* **336** (1990) 65-71.

[3]   Gruppo Italiano per lo Studio della Sopravvivenza nell'Infarto Miocardico. GISSI-3: effects of lisinopril and transdermal glyceryl trinitrate singly and together on 6-week mortality and ventricular function after acute myocardial infarction. *Lancet* **343** (1994) 1115-1122.

[4]   GISSI-Prevenzione Investigators. Dietary supplementation with n-3 polyunsaturated fatty acids and vitamin E after myocardial infarction: results of the GISSI-Prevenzione trial. Gruppo Italiano per lo Studio della Sopravvivenza nell'Infarto Miocardico. *Lancet* **354** (1999) 447-455.

[5]   L. Hansson, A. Zanchetti, S.G. Carruthers *et al.* Effects of intensive blood-pressure lowering and low-dose aspirin in patients with hypertension: principal results of the Hypertension Optimal Treatment (HOT) randomised trial. *Lancet* **351** (1998) 1755-1762.

[6]   M.L. Burr, A.M. Fehily, J.F. Gilbert *et al.* Effects of changes in fat, fish, and fibre intakes on death and myocardial reinfarction: diet and reinfarction trial (DART). *Lancet* **2** (1989) 757-761.

[7]   R. Marchioli. Treatment with n-3 polyunsaturated fatty acids after myocardial infarction: results of GISSI-prevenzione trial. *Eur. Heart J. Suppl.* **3** (2001) D85-D97.

[8]   D. Wood, G. De Backer, O. Faergeman *et al.* Prevention of coronary heart disease in clinical practice. Recommendations of the Second Joint Task Force of European and other Societies on coronary prevention. *Eur. Heart J.* **19** (1998) 1434-1503.

[9]   Scandinavian Simvastatin Survival Study Group. Randomised trial of cholesterol lowering in 4444 patients with coronary heart disease: the Scandinavian Simvastatin Survival Study (4S). *Lancet* **344** (1994) 1383-1389.

[10] J. Shepherd, S.M. Cobbe, I. Ford *et al.* Prevention of coronary heart disease with pravastatin in men with hypercholesterolemia. West of Scotland Coronary Prevention Study Group. *N. Engl. J. Med.* **333** (1995) 1301-1307.

[11] F.M. Sacks, M.A. Pfeffer, L.A. Moyé *et al.* The effect of pravastatin on coronary events after myocardial infarction in patients with average cholesterol levels. Cholesterol and Recurrent Events Trial Investigators. *N. Engl. J. Med.* **335** (1996) 1001-1009.

[12] LIPID Study Group. Prevention of cardiovascular events and death with pravastatin in patients with coronary heart disease and a broad range of initial cholesterol levels. The Long-Term Intervention with Pravastatin in Ischaemic Disease (LIPID) Study Group. *N. Engl. J. Med.* **339** (1998) 1349-1357.

[13] R.P. Byington, J.W. Jukema, J.T. Salonen *et al.* Reduction in cardiovascular events during pravastatin therapy. Pooled analysis of clinical events of the Pravastatin Atherosclerosis Intervention Program. *Circulation* **92** (1995) 2419-2425.

[14] D.W. Nilsen, G. Albrektsen, K. Landmark *et al.* Effects of a high-dose concentrate of n-3 fatty acids or corn oil introduced early after an acute myocardial infarction on serum triacylglycerol and HDL cholesterol. *Am. J. Clin. Nutr.* **74** (2001) 50-56.

[15] D.W. Nilsen and W.S. Harris. N-3 Fatty acids and cardiovascular disease. *Am. J. Clin. Nutr.* **79** (2004) 166.

[16] R. Marchioli, F. Barzi, E. Bomba *et al.* Early protection against sudden death by n-3 polyunsaturated fatty acids after myocardial infarction: time-course analysis of the results of Gruppo Italiano per lo Studio della Sopravvivenza nell'Infarto Miocardico (GISSI)-Prevenzione. *Circulation* **105** (2002) 1897-1903.

[17] E. Lonn, J. Bosch, S. Yusuf *et al.* for the HOPE and HOPE-TOO Trial Investigators. Effects of long-term vitamin E supplementation on cardiovascular events and cancer: a randomized controlled trial. *JAMA* **293** (2005) 1338-1347.

[18] Heart Protection Study Collaborative group. MRC/BHF Heart Protection Study of antioxidant vitamin supplementation in 20,536 high-risk individuals: a randomised placebo-controlled trial. *Lancet* **360** (2002) 23-33.

[19]   D.P. Vivekananthan, M.S. Penn, S.K. Sapp *et al.* Use of antioxidant vitamins for the prevention of cardiovascular disease: meta-analysis of randomised trials. *Lancet* **361** (2003) 2017-2023.

[20]   I.M. Lee, N.R. Cook, J.M. Gaziano *et al.* Vitamin E in the primary prevention of cardiovascular disease and cancer: the Women's Health Study: a randomized controlled trial. *JAMA* **294** (2005) 56-65.

[21]   M. Boaz, S. Smetana, T. Weinstein *et al.* Secondary prevention with antioxidants of cardiovascular disease in endstage renal disease (SPACE): randomised placebo-controlled trial. *Lancet* **356** (2000) 1213-1218.

[22]   M. Studer, M. Briel, B. Leimenstoll *et al.* Effect of different antilipidemic agents and diets on mortality: a systematic review. *Arch. Intern. Med.* **165** (2005) 725-730.

[23]   J.X. Kang and A. Leaf. Antiarrhythmic effects of polyunsaturated fatty acids. Recent studies. *Circulation* **94** (1996) 1774-1780.

[24]   I.H. Rosenberg. Fish - food to calm the heart. *N. Engl. J. Med.* **346** (2002) 1102-1103.

[25]   A. Leaf and J.X. Kang. Prevention of cardiac sudden death by N-3 fatty acids: a review of the evidence. *J. Intern. Med.* **240** (1996) 5-12.

[26]   J.X. Kang and A. Leaf. Prevention of fatal cardiac arrhythmias by polyunsaturated fatty acids. *Am. J. Clin. Nutr.* **71** (2000) 202S-207S.

[27]   J.X. Kang and A. Leaf. Evidence that free polyunsaturated fatty acids modify Na^+ channels by directly binding to the channel proteins. *Proc. Natl. Acad. Sci. U.S.A.* **93** (1996) 3542-3546.

[28]   H. Hallaq, T.W. Smith, A. Leaf. Modulation of dihydropyridine-sensitive calcium channels in heart cells by fish oil fatty acids. *Proc. Natl. Acad. Sci. U.S.A.* **89** (1992) 1760-1764.

[29]   R. Marchioli, F. Avanzini, F. Barzi *et al.* Assessment of absolute risk of death after myocardial infarction by use of multiple-risk-factor assessment equations: GISSI-Prevenzione mortality risk chart. *Eur. Heart J.* **22** (2001) 2085-2103.

[30]   A. Macchia, G. Levantesi, M.G. Franzosi *et al.* Left ventricular systolic dysfunction, total mortality, and sudden death in patients with myocardial infarction treated with n-3 polyunsaturated fatty acids. *Eur. J. Heart Fail.* **7** (2005) 904-909.

[31]   R. De Caterina and G. Basta. n-3 fatty acids and the inflammatory response - biological background. *Eur. Heart J. Suppl.* **3** (2001) D42-D49.

[32]   H. Rupp, M. Turcani, T. Ohkubo *et al.* Dietary linolenic acid-mediated increase in vascular prostacyclin formation. *Mol. Cell. Biochem.* **162** (1996) 59-64.

[33]   A.J. Brown and D.C. Roberts. Fish and fish oil intake: effect on haematological variables related to cardiovascular disease. *Thromb. Res.* **64** (1991) 169-178.

[34]   K.H. Weylandt and J.X. Kang. Rethinking lipid mediators. *Lancet* **366** (2005) 618-620.

[35]   F. Barzi, M. Woodward, R.M. Marfisi *et al.* Mediterranean diet and all-causes mortality after myocardial infarction: results from the GISSI-Prevenzione trial. *Eur. J. Clin. Nutr.* **57** (2003) 604-611.

[36]   N. Kimura and A. Keys. Coronary heart disease in seven countries. X. Rural southern Japan. *Circulation* **41** (1970) I101-I112.

[37]   M. de Lorgeril and P. Salen. Diet as preventive medicine in cardiology. *Curr. Opin. ardiol.* **15** (2000) 364-370.

[38]   A.R. Ness and J.W. Powles. Fruit and vegetables, and cardiovascular disease: a review. *Int. J. Epidemiol.* **26** (1997) 1-13.

[39]   R.M. Krauss, R.H. Eckel, B. Howard *et al.* AHA Dietary Guidelines: revision 2000: A statement for healthcare professionals from the Nutrition Committee of the American Heart Association. *Circulation* **102** (2000) 2284-2299.

[40]   G. Levantesi, A. Macchia, R. Marfisi *et al.* Metabolic syndrome and risk of cardiovascular events after myocardial infarction. *J. Am. Coll. Cardiol.* **46** (2005) 277-283.

[41]   M.G. Franzosi, M. Brunetti, R. Marchioli *et al.* Cost-effectiveness of n-3 polyunsaturated fatty acids (PUFA) after myocardial infarction: results from Gruppo Italiano per lo Studio della Sopravvivenza nell'Infarto (GISSI)-Prevenzione Trial. *Pharmacoeconomics* **19** (2001) 411-420.

Cardiovascular Benefits of Omega-3 Polyunsaturated Fatty Acids
B. Maisch and R. Oelze (Eds.)
IOS Press, 2006

Prevention of Cardiovascular Diseases and Highly Concentrated n-3 Polyunsaturated Fatty Acids (PUFAs)

Heinz S. Weber, Dzevair Selimi and Gustav Huber
*1ˢᵗ Medical Department, SMZ-Ost/Danube Hospital, Langobardenstrasse 122, A-1220
Vienna, Austria*

Abstract. 30 years ago the observation of a lower incidence of cardiovascular diseases in Inuits (Eskimos) was related to the higher fish consumption when compared to the residual Danish population. Clinical studies confirmed this finding. It was explained by the higher content of polyunsaturated fatty acids (PUFA) in fish, especially of omega-3 PUFAs. Experimental studies in cell cultures and also in animals with and without infarction models verified the anti-arrhythmic effect of omega-3 PUFAs among other possible contributing factors when compared to other fatty acids. In clinical studies a significant reduction (ca. 40%) of sudden cardiac deaths (SCD) could be found in patients after an acute myocardial infarction (AMI), if they were treated with at least 1 g omega-3 PUFAs daily, either by consumption of fish twice weekly or of a highly purified preparation omega-3 PUFAs in capsules. These findings led to recommendations of the American Heart Association and the European Society of Cardiology (ESC) to a higher fish consumption and/or the daily intake of 1 g O-3 PUFAs for primary and especially for secondary prevention of cardiovascular diseases. The much fewer side-effects, and the standardised dosage on one hand and the negative effect of the sometimes higher mercury content of fish make the intake of omega-3 PUFAs as capsules the better choice.

Keywords. Cardiovascular disease, fatty acids, sudden death, myocardial infarction, O-3 PUFAs

Introduction

One of the main contemporary challenges in medicine is to reduce the global burden of cardiovascular diseases (CVD). CVDs are responsible for 10% of DALY's (disability-adjusted life-years), which represent the global burden of CVD, in low- and middle-income countries and for 18% in high-income countries [1]. An estimated 17 million people die of CVDs, i.e. about 30% of all deaths, 13% are related to coronary heart disease (CHD) and 10% to stroke [1].

The fight against CVDs includes preventive methods and treatment strategies. The latter are more spectacular (e.g. PTCA, stents, bypass surgery) and popular with patients (drugs, e.g. "lifestyle drugs"). Cardiologists and cardiac surgeons offering these methods became contemporary medical heroes, because of their nearly immediate effects: pain relief, improvement of left ventricular function (LVF), prevention of myocardial infarction, avoiding of disability and reduction of mortality.

Prevention needs a continuous effort of the patient for physical exercise and a change in nutrition habits, no matter whether we consider primary, secondary or tertiary prevention. Prevention and a new lifestyle reduce, what many people consider their "quality of life" (QOL): stop smoking, 30 minutes daily exercise, healthy food etc. became the main preventive messages for daily life. Frequently it includes also a regular intake of tablets that are neither a pain-killer nor do they make the person feel better and which may have some side-effects as well. In general prevention costs money, the general population can be hardly convinced of its value and results can only be seen after several years. Therefore prevention is not really very popular.

To change this attitude was a challenge, which was brought to the public: the realisation of CVD prevention programs in the communities. More and more political leaders and also a larger proportion of the population can now be convinced from the tremendous importance of prevention. This is a prerequisite, if we are to improve our QOL, to live longer and to reduce disabilities due to CVD events [2].

Several international and national scientific organisations published their recommendations and their guidelines on the prevention in CVD based on epidemiological evidence and studies published in recent peer-reviewed publications. They represent today's medical evidence. Among them are the American Heart Association (AHA) [3,4] and the European Society of Cardiology (ESC) [5,6]. Based on these ESC-guidelines and on the EU Council Conclusions on Heart Health [7] the EU Commission for Health and Consumer Protection published together with the ESC the "Luxembourg Declaration on Prevention of CVD" in June 2005 [8], which summarizes and simplifies for the public understanding the basics of prevention: no smoking, at least 30 minutes daily physical activity, healthy food choices, blood pressure below 140/90, blood cholesterol <5 mmol/l (200 mg/dl). Furthermore a "European Charter on Heart Health" will be worked out and should be published in 2006 under the Finish EU presidency.

Among the above mentioned recommendations nutrition plays a major part in teaching prevention, especially the quality and quantity of daily fat intake [5]. Food should be varied and energy intake must be adjusted to maintain an ideal body weight [6]. Food consumption should be based on fruits and vegetables, whole grain, cereals and bread, low fat dairy products, fish and lean meat [6]. Total fat intake should not exceed 30% of total energy intake, whereby oily fish and polyunsaturated omega-3 fatty acids (O-3 PUFAs) have particular protective properties [6]. Saturated fats should not exceed one-third of total fat intake [6].

This contribution will discuss possible mechanisms of omega-3 PUFAs for preventing CVD, especially reducing sudden cardiac death (SCD) and delineate why PUFAs became part of the AHA- and ESC-prevention guidelines.

1. The Very Beginning of a Suspected Relation between PUFAs and CVDs

Greenland Eskimos have a low incidence of CVDs. The Eskimo meals have a much higher content of omega-3 PUFAs when compared to the eating habits of the residual Danish population [9]. The obvious cause was the higher fish consumption of Eskimos, especially the Inuits, a tribe among them. Therefore fish-rich nutrition was called the "Inuit-diet". Further epidemiologic studies demonstrated variable results: some could demonstrate the cardioprotective effect of fish consumption, other studies were negative [10,11] or inconsistent [12,13]. Over all modest fish intake will lead to a 50% decrease in the risk of sudden cardiac death (SCD), but not in the risk of non-SCD or myocardial infarction [14,15]. Since fish is rich in omega-3 PUFAs, the conclusion was that these PUFAs are responsible for the low CVD incidence of the Eskimos and also for the SCD risk reduction [16].

Meanwhile more than 11 controlled or randomized clinical trials (RCTs) deal with the secondary prevention in coronary heart disease by omega-3 PUFAs and were summarized as a meta-analysis [17].

2. Possible Mechanisms of Omega-3 PUFAs Preventing CVD

Several effects of omega-3 PUFAs could be demonstrated in *in vitro* and *in vivo* trials [18,19]:

- Retarded growth of the atherosclerotic plaque [18,20-24]:
    - Reduction of adhesion molecule expression;
    - Reduction of platelet-derived growth factor;
    - Anti-inflammatory properties;
- Promotion of NO-induced endothelial relaxation;
- Antithrombogenic effects [25,26];
- Reduced susceptibility of the heart to ventricular arrhythmias;
- Hypotriglyceridaemic effects (fasting and postprandial), i.e. lowering triglycerides;
- Mild hypotensive effects.

Anti-arrhythmic Effects of O-3 PUFAs in Experimental Studies

In the middle of the past century, around 1950, it was observed that free fatty acids liberated during acute ischaemia led to ventricular arrhythmias and SCD [27]. 25 years later a preventive effect on ventricular arrhythmias in humans was considered with fish oil intake [28]. In a rabbit heart model saturated fatty acids lowered the fibrillation threshold, whereas PUFAs increased it [29]. This was one possible explanation for their anti-arrhythmic effect. Feeding rats during an experimental acute myocardial infarction (AMI) with vegetable (PUFAs) or olive oil (monounsaturated fatty acids) the ventricular fibrillation rate could be reduced by 70% in the PUFA-group [30]. Ventricular fibrillation, induced by an ischaemic stress did never appear again after i.v. injection of PUFAs in a dog model [31].
These and other cell and animal experiments led to the current hypotheses of the anti-arrhythmic actions of omega-3 PUFAs [27]:

- Hyperpolarisation of the resting potential of the myocardial cells with an increase of the fibrillation threshold. A higher stimulus will be necessary to induce ventricular fibrillation.
- Inhibition of the fast, voltage-dependent sodium channels of the action potential (phase-0 depolarisation). This is important especially in acute myocardial infection, when myocytes in the periphery of the ischaemic zone become hyperexcitable. These cells are the typical substrate for life-threatening arrhythmias (VT, VF) and SCD. PUFAs will slip the Na-channels of these hyperpolarised cells quicker into the "resting inactivation" and by this mechanism prevent these arrhythmias.
- Inhibition of the L-type calcium currents, which has a preventive effect on the delayed after-potential discharges caused by excessive Ca-fluctuations. Delayed after-potentials are an underlying mechanism for the induction of polymorphic ventricular tachycardias ("Torsade de Pointes").
- Prolongation of phase-4 repolarisation.

These experimental findings are the basis for the explanation, how omega-3 PUFAs may prevent sudden cardiac death.

3. Omega-3 PUFAs and Sudden Cardiac Death (SCD)

In the period before we became aware of the anti-arrhythmic effect of PUFAs, the first clinical study, which investigated the beneficial effects in secondary prevention of myocardial infarction by the advice on fish and fibre intake was DART [32]. After two years follow-up a 29% mortality reduction could be observed in the group with a high weekly fish intake, the consumption being at least 200-400g twice a week. No differences could be found with respect to fat and fibre intake.

The next secondary prevention trial in AMI compared in a randomized and prospective, single blinded manner the value of a Mediterranean-diet, which was rich in PUFAs, with a usual diet [33]. The study, expected for a 5-year follow-up, had to be stopped much earlier, because of the beneficial effects of the Mediterranean-diet group: the mortality and the reinfarction rates were significantly (p<0,001) lower in the group with an high amount of PUFA intake.

The GISSI-trial [34] compared in a prospective, randomized manner 4 different groups of post-AMI prevention strategies: PUFAs alone, daily 1 g, Vitamin E alone, both combined and a control group. All participating patients had the usual post-AMI medication, predominantly aspirin, beta-blockers, ACE-inhibitors and statins. The latter were given in the beginning not so frequently, since they came up later in the trial. As a consequence of the former trial [33] a Mediterranean diet was recommended for all participants. The data demonstrated a significant positive effect on the primary end-point especially in the first post-AMI year only in the groups receiving PUFAs when compared to the control group and to the patient cohort receiving Vitamin E. This primary end-point was death, non-fatal AMI and stroke, which were reduced by 15%. The risk of death was lowered by 20%, the risk of cardiovascular death by 30%.

The study was criticised because it had only a control and not a placebo group. A further criticism was that statins were used in only few patients and, when given, this was only at the end of the study.

SCD was not an end-point of the study. But it became quickly obvious that SCD was the major cause of death in the study. Therefore the study was reanalysed with special emphasis on SCDs [35]. A reduction of SCD could be found in the same groups as in the original results [34] of about 40%, which was the most impressive change in the entire GISSI-Prevenzione trial. It was concluded that the lower all-cause mortality and also the reduction of cardiovascular mortality was predominantly related to the reduction of sudden cardiac death.

The fundamental finding of the GISSI-P trial was that the reduction of SCD in the post-AMI period was independent from lipid-lowering and it was due to taking daily 1 g omega-3 PUFAs. Remarkably it could be reproduced by other studies [14,15,36].

In an retrospective analysis of the Physicians' Health Study [37], with a 17-year follow-up for the measurement of omega-3 PUFAs blood levels, the SCD risk reduction was 81%. This was the highest risk reduction found in any PUFA study ever published.

This SCD risk reduction of omega-3 PUFAs was analysed using a questionnaire in 45.722 men free of CVD over a period of 14 years [38].

In a meta-analysis of prospective cohort studies between 1966-2003 including 11 studies with 13 cohorts and 222.364 individuals with a mean follow-up of 12 years the authors concluded that each 20 g/d-fish intake lowers the CHD mortality risk by 7% (p=0,03) [39].

The prolongation of the QTc-interval is a predictor of an increased risk for life-threatening arrhythmias and SCD. The influence of dietary linolic acids (LA) on the QTc was investigated prospectively in 3.642 subjects without any AMI, hypertrophy, pacemaker and with normal QRS width. In a multivariate model the QTc was inversely related to the LA intake especially in men. It was concluded that a higher intake of dietary LA might be associated with a reduced risk of abnormally prolonged repolarisation [40].

In recent trials the anti-arrhythmic effect of omega-3 PUFAs was evaluated in patients with implantable defibrillators (ICD), whereas the ICD discharges are compared in a randomized manner between a PUFA-diet group and other groups, e.g. diet with olive oil [41]. The results did not show a significant reduction of the expected events (SCD, ICD discharges, VT or VF in the -EKGs) after one year in the PUFA-group, but the authors concluded nevertheless "…that for individuals at high risk for fatal ventricular arrhythmias regular daily ingestions of fish oil fatty acids may significantly reduce potentially fatal arrhythmias." [41].

Also in supraventricular arrhythmias a protective effect of n-3 PUFAs could be found in the incidence of paroxysmal atrial fibrillation in the postoperative period after CABG surgery [42].

There is increasing evidence that omega-3 PUFAs have a beneficial effect in the post-AMI period on mortality, especially on SCD, which is predominately related to life-threatening arrhythmias. Experimental models can explain the anti-arrhythmic and preventive effects of PUFAs. But a convincing result of at least one prospective RCT to prove the hypotheses that PUFAs reduce an elevated SCD risk is still missing today.

Nevertheless there are enough scientific data demonstrating that PUFAs are to be included in several CHD prevention guidelines.

4. Fish versus Highly Purified Omega-3 PUFAs as Pharmacon

4.1. The Essential PUFAs

Food lipids consist of three major classes, which are based on the number of double bonds between carbon atoms: the saturated fatty acids (FA), the monounsaturated FA and the polyunsaturated FA (Figure 1) [43]. In the "Seven Countries" study only the mainly intake of saturated FA was associated with a significantly higher mortality after 10 respectively 25 years of control [44]. The sources of saturated FA are animal products (i.e. meat and dairy products), butter, lard and should be reduced if not avoided in all CHD preventive efforts [3-8]. It increases the LDL cholesterol level in contrast to PUFAs.

The unsaturated FA cannot be produced in our body and therefore are called "essential" FA. Mono- and polyunsaturated FA are in several oils, fish, nuts, sunflower etc. (Figure 1).

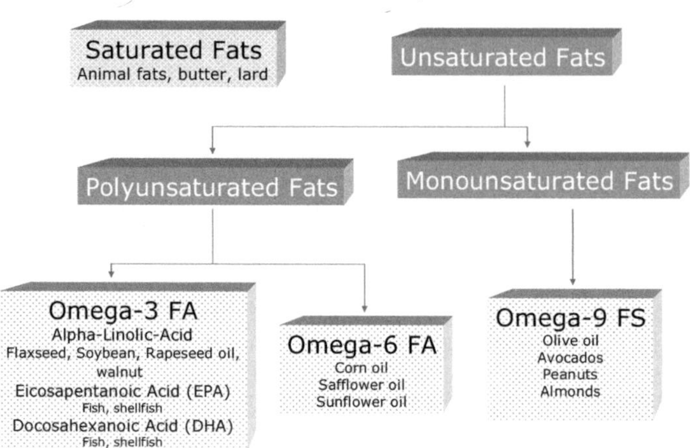

Figure 1. Fats and fatty acids [modified 43].

EPA and DHA are physiologically the most important long-chain omega-3 PUFAs, which were synthesized under the support of desaturases and elongases from alpha-linolenic acid, the shortest omega-3 PUFA (Figure 2). Sources of O-3 PUFAs generally are marine vertebrates. Essential FAs are accumulated in the phospholipids of the cell membrane especially in the cells of the brain, heart and testes. They are responsible for the growth and the optimal function of these organs mentioned [27].

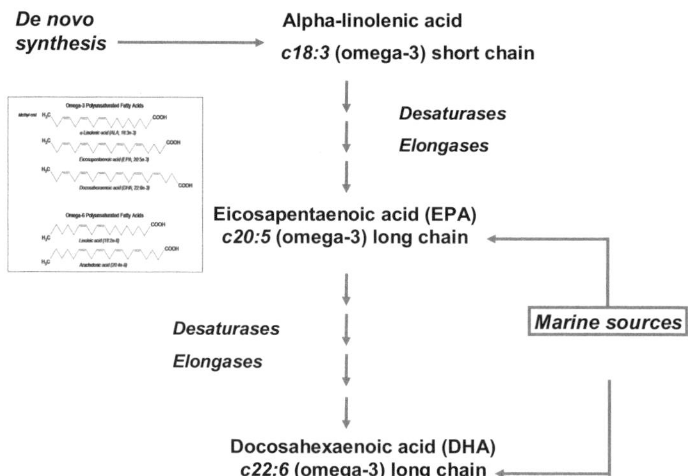

Figure 2. Biosynthesis of O-3 PUFAs.

4.2. Marine Sources of Essential Fatty Acids

De Lorgeril investigated the content of the different omega-3 PUFAs in several sorts of fish. He could demonstrate a tremendous dependency of the amount of PUFAs from the season, the localisation of the fishing area and the cooking preparation (raw or cooked) [16]. The highest content of total omega-3 PUFAs could be found in the Atlantic mackerel during the autumn season, but only in raw conditions. The omega-3 PUFA content was estimated by 6,57 g/100g fish.

The consumption of fish does not only have the above mentioned advantages, but may also have side-effects related to their mercury content. A possible relationship between the mercury level in the toenails and coronary heart diseases (CHD) were investigated in a case-control study including more than 33.000 individuals consuming frequently fish [45]. A close correlation between the mercury levels and the amount of fish consumption could be found, but no significant correlation to the risk of CHD, although a marginal interdependence was not be ruled out by the authors [45]. Another case-control study compared the mercury toenail content of 684 men with AMI and 724 men with no evidence of CHD. The authors found a direct association with the risk of AMI and the mercury toenail content. They concluded that the mercury content may diminish the cardio protective effect of O-3 PUFAs [46].

Therefore in 2004 the FDA published an advice for women, who might become pregnant or who are pregnant, for nursing mothers and for young children: they should not eat fish with high mercury content, which are shark, swordfish, king mackerel and tilefish [47]. The FDA recommends 12 ounces (i.e. 2 average meals, each 180 g) a week of fish and shellfish, which are lower in mercury, especially shrimp, canned light tuna fish, salmon, pollock and catfish [47].

4.3. Highly Purified Omega-3 PUFAs as 1g-capsules

Beyond the recommendation for more fish meals and in view of the heavy metal contents of fish a capsule consisting of 1g highly purified omega-3 PUFAs was developed, which were well-tolerated. The content of omega-3 PUFAs was 90%, 46% EPA, 38% DHA and 6% other O-3 PUFAs [48]. This capsule (OMACOR®) was used in the GISSI-P trial [34,35] and also in other upcoming trials especially because of the convenience of the drug intake and the constant dosage. Furthermore the plasma level can be increased more easily using capsules than eating fish with unsure contents of fatty acids. Here also it could be shown, that an increase in omega-3 PUFA levels decreases the risk of SCD [37]. The daily intake of 1g highly purified O-3 PUFA (OMACOR®) raised the plasma level from 2,9% to 6% which was associated with a marked cardiac protection [49].

4.4. Side-Effects of Omega-3 PUFAs

The risk of side-effects from the intake of omega-3 PUFAs is generally very low. Side-effects were analysed in detail in an AHA-Scientific Statement [18] and are clearly dose-dependent.

Up to 1 g omega-3 PUFAs per day, which is the recommended dosage for CHD prevention (secondary and primary) and prevention of SCD, side-effects are considered either very low or low.

If a higher dosage (2-4 g/d) is needed, especially if PUFAs are used for lowering triglycerides, side-effects occur more frequently and become less tolerated, especially gastrointestinal upset, fishy aftertaste and worsening of glycaemia in patients with impaired glucose tolerance and diabetes [18].

The occurrence of gastrointestinal upsets is classified as very low when 1 g/d are given and moderate when >1 g/d is administered.

Clinical bleeding is also a possible side-effect under PUFA medication, but is a rare condition and ranges from very low to low. Fishy aftertaste occurs frequently in higher dosages, but the occurrence is low if the usual dose of 1 g/d is used. As mentioned above worsening of glycaemia relates to the PUFA-dosage as well as to the glucose intolerance of the patient. LDL cholesterol can rise with a higher dosage usually only in patients with hypertriglyceridaemia, in whom PUFAs are added to statins for triglyceride-lowering [18].

5. CVD Prevention Using Omega-3 PUFAs: Guidelines and Recommendations

The need of essential fatty acids for daily life, the negative effect of saturated fatty acids, the proven preventive effect of omega-3 PUFAs and the reduction of SCD-mortality risk with a favourable drug profile with only few and without any life-threatening side-effects are the reasons, why the intake of O-3 PUFAs are recommended in several prevention guidelines:

The American Heart Association (AHA)-Guidelines recommend for CHD prevention [3,18]:
- In patients without documented CHD without infarction (primary prevention) they recommend to eat a variety of (preferable oily) fish at least twice a week. Furthermore oils and foods rich in alpha-linolenic acid should be preferred, i.e. flaxseed, canola, soybean oils, and walnuts.
- In patients with documented CHD after infarction (secondary and tertiary prevention) at least 1 g of EPA and DHA per day should be taken, preferably from oily fish. Supplements could be considered in consultation with the physician.
- In patients who need triglyceride-lowering 2-4 g of EPA and DHA per day will be recommended, which can be provided only as capsules under the physician's care.

The primary recommendation of the AHA is a dietary, food-based approach to increase omega-3 PUFA intake. But they were also aware that the necessary dosage may be greater than what could be achieved by fish intake alone. Therefore other supplements should be considered. The AHA concludes that "the availability of high-quality omega-3 PUFA supplements, free of contaminants, is an important prerequisite to their extensive use" [18].

The European Guidelines for CV prevention [5,6] recommend under the title "make healthy food choices",
- that total fat intake should be restricted to 30% of energy intake,
- that intake of saturated fatty acids should not exceed a third of total fat intake,
- that the intake of cholesterol should be less than 300 mg/d,
- and that oily fish and omega-3 fatty acids seem to have particular protective effects.

In secondary prevention of CHD the administration of 1 g omega-3 PUFAs daily is classified as indication class 1, which means there is a general agreement and evidence to do so. Also the evidence level is classified as evidence B, because only one prospective RCT is at present available to show the protective effect in post-AMI patients on SCD [5,6].

The daily intake of at least 1 g of omega-3 PUFAs, either in form of food or as highly purified capsules is recommended by both international organisations, the AHA and the ESC. Especially in secondary AMI prevention this safe medication should never be withheld to any patient.

6. Summary

During the past 30 years more than 7.000 reports including nearly 900 clinical trials were published related to fish oil and/or omega-3 PUFAs [50]. All these trials, which could be discussed in this contribution only selectively, contributed to the present view of the utmost necessity of the essential fatty acids, their actions on a cellular basis and in *in vitro* studies. Clinical observations of a lower incidence of CVDs, comparing in the past century the nutrition behaviours of the Inuits with a higher amount of fish and so for omega-3 PUFAs with the general Danish population, was the beginning for many new experiments and ideas.

Clinical trials verified the preventive effects of omega-3 PUFAs on SCD in the post-AMI period, which was predominately arrhythmogenic. This anti-arrhythmic effect of the PUFAs could be explained by experiments in cell and animal models and will be extended obviously also to supraventricular arrhythmias (atrial fibrillation).

Several fish meals a week is a strongly recommended diet, but has the disadvantage of heavy metal pollution of many of the marine PUFA sources. Therefore the artificial, but highly purified omega-3 PUFA capsules with a standardised content and nearly no side-effects should be used as an alternative or better as additive to the healthy nutrition.

7. Conclusion

Who will argue against the highly recommended daily 1 g omega-3 PUFAs as an important and safe tool in secondary, but also in primary CVD prevention? There is much more benefits than harm, if ever, and little costs. Fish or highly purified omega-3 PUFA capsules could and should be recommended to everybody.

References

[1]   J. Mackay and G. Mensah. The atlas of heart disease and stroke. *WHO* (2004). ISBN 9241562765.
[2]   D.A. Wood, K. Kotseva, C. Jennings *et al*. EUROACTION: A European Society of Cardiology demonstration project in preventive cardiology: A cluster randomised controlled trial of a multi-disciplinary preventive cardiology programme for coronary patients, asymptomatic high risk individuals and their families. Summary of design, methodology and outcomes. *Eur. Heart J. Suppl.* **6** (2004) J3-J15.
[3]   T.A. Pearson, S.N. Blair, S.R. Daniels *et al*. AHA Guidelines for primary prevention of cardiovascular disease and stroke: 2002 update. *Circulation* **106** (2002) 388-391.
[4]   M.A. Williams, J.L. Fleg, P.A. Ades *et al*. Secondary prevention of coronary heart disease in the elderly (with emphasis on patients > or =75 years of age): an American Heart Association scientific statement from the Council on Clinical Cardiology Subcommittee on Exercise, Cardiac Rehabilitation, and Prevention. *Circulation* **105** (2002) 1735-1743.
[5]   G. De Backer, E. Ambrosioni, K. Borch-Johnsen *et al*. European guidelines on cardiovascular disease prevention in clinical practice. *Eur. J. Cardiovasc. Prev. Rehab.* **10** (2003) S1-S10.
[6]   G. De Backer, E. Ambrosioni, K. Borch-Johnsen *et al*. European guidelines on cardiovascular disease prevention in clinical practice. *Eur. Heart J.* **24** (2003) 1601-1610.
[7]   EU Council. Conclusions on Heart Health, 2586th Council Meeting Employment, Social Policy, Health and Consumer Affairs, 1-2. Luxembourg (June 2004).

[8]   http://www.escardio.org/NR/rdonlyres/97677661-EEA7-4AA3-81C3-
       1B59C2D6A542/0/LuxembourgDeclaration.pdf

[9]   H.O. Bang, J. Dyerberg, H.M. Sinclair. The composition of the Eskimo food in north western
       Greenland. *Am. J. Clin. Nutr.* **33** (1980) 2657-2661.

[10]   A. Ascherio, E.B. Rimm, M.J. Stampfer *et al.* Dietary intake of marine n-3 fatty acids, fish intake, and
       the risk of coronary disease among men. *N. Engl. J. Med.* **332** (1995) 977-982.

[11]   M.C. Morris, J.E. Manson, B. Rosner *et al.* Fish consumption and cardiovascular disease in the
       physicians' health study: a prospective study. *Am. J. Epidemiol.* **142** (1995) 166-175.

[12]   M.L. Daviglus, J. Stamler, A.J. Orencia *et al.* Fish consumption and the 30-year risk of fatal
       myocardial infarction. *N. Engl. J. Med.* **336** (1997) 1046-1053.

[13]   C.M. Oomen, E.J. Feskens, L. Rasanen *et al.* Fish consumption and coronary heart disease mortality in
       Finland, Italy, and The Netherlands. *Am. J. Epidemiol.* **151** (2000) 999-1006.

[14]   D.S. Siscovick, T.E. Raghunathan, I. King *et al.* Dietary intake and cell membrane levels of long-chain
       n-3 polyunsaturated fatty acids and the risk of primary cardiac arrest. *JAMA* **274** (1995) 1363-1367.

[15]   C.M. Albert, C.H. Hennekens, C.J. O'Donnell *et al.* Fish consumption and risk of sudden cardiac death.
       JAMA **279** (1998) 23-28.

[16]   M. de Lorgeril and P. Salen. Fish and N-3 fatty acids for the prevention and treatment of coronary
       heart disease: nutrition is not pharmacology. *Am. J. Med.* **112** (2002) 316-319.

[17]   H.C. Bucher, P. Hengstler, C. Schindler *et al.* N-3 polyunsaturated fatty acids in coronary heart
       disease: a meta-analysis of randomized controlled trials. *Am. J. Med.* **112** (2002) 298-304.

[18]   P.M. Kris-Etherton, W.S. Harris, L.J. Appel. Fish consumption, fish oil, omega-3 fatty acids and
       cardiovascular disease. *Circulation* **106** (2002) 2747-2757.

[19]   W.E. Connor. Importance of n-3 fatty acids in health and disease. *Am. J. Clin. Nutr.* **71** (2000) 171S-
       175S.

[20]   R. De Caterina and P. Libby. Control of endothelial leukocyte adhesion molecules by fatty acids.
       Lipids **31** (1996) S57-S63.

[21]   R. De Caterina, J.K. Liao, P. Libby. Fatty acid modulation of endothelial activation. *Am. J. Clin. Nutr.*
       71 (2000) 213S-223S.

[22]   Y. Abe, B. El-Masri, K.T. Kimball *et al.* Soluble cell adhesion molecules in hypertriglyceridemia and
       potential significance on monocyte adhesion. *Arterioscler. Thromb. Vasc. Biol.* **18** (1998) 723-731.

[23]   I. Seljeflot, H. Arnesen, I.R. Brude *et al.* Effects of omega-3 fatty acids and/or antioxidants on
       endothelial cell markers. *Eur. J. Clin. Invest.* **28** (1998) 629-635.

[24]   S. Endres and C. von Schacky. n-3 polyunsaturated fatty acids and human cytokine synthesis. *Curr.*
       Opin. Lipidol. **7** (1996) 48-52.

[25]   J.J. Agren, S. Vaisanen, O. Hanninen *et al.* Hemostatic factors and platelet aggregation after a fish-
       enriched diet or fish oil or docosahexaenoic acid supplementation. *Prostaglandins Leukot. Essent.*
       Fatty Acids **57** (1997) 419-421.

[26]   T.A. Mori, L.J. Beilin, V. Burke *et al.* Interactions between dietary fat, fish, and fish oils and their
       effects on platelet function in men at risk of cardiovascular disease. *Arterioscler. Thromb. Vasc. Biol.*
       17 (1997) 279-286.

[27]   A. Leaf, J.X. Kang, Y.F. Xiao *et al.* Clinical prevention of sudden cardiac death by n-3
       polyunsaturated fatty acids and mechanism of prevention of arrhythmias by n-3 fish oils. *Circulation*
       107 (2003) 2646-2652.

[28]   S. Gudbjarnason and J. Hallgrimsson. The role of myocardial membrane lipids in the development of
       cardiac necrosis. *Acta Med. Scand. Suppl.* **587** (1976) 17-27.

[29]   M.F. Murnaghan. Effects of fatty acids on the ventricular arrhythmia threshold in the isolated heart of
       the rabbit. *Br. J. Pharmacol.* **73** (1981) 909-915.

[30]   P.L. McLennan, M.Y. Abeywardena, J.S. Charnock. Dietary fish oil prevents ventricular fibrillation
       following coronary artery occlusion and reperfusion. *Am. Heart J.* **116** (1988) 709-717.

[31]   G.E. Billman, J.X. Kang, A. Leaf. Prevention of sudden cardiac death by dietary pure omega-3
       polyunsaturated fatty acids in dogs. *Circulation* **99** (1999) 2452-2457.

[32]   M.L. Burr, A.M. Fehily, J.F. Gilbert *et al.* Effect of changes in fat, fish and fibre intakes on death and
       myocardial reinfarction: diet and reinfarction trial (DART). *Lancet* **2** (1989) 757-761.

[33]   M. de Lorgeril, P. Salen, J.L. Martin *et al.* Mediterranean diet, traditional risk factors, and the rate of
       cardiovascular complications after myocardial infarction: final report of the Lyon Diet Heart Study.
       Circulation **99** (1999) 779-785.

[34]   GISSI-Prevenzione Investigators. Dietary supplementation with n-3 polyunsaturated fatty acids and
       vitamin E after myocardial infarction: results of the GISSI-Prevenzione trial. Gruppo Italiano per lo
       Studio della Sopravvivenza nell'Infarto miocardico. *Lancet* **354** (1999) 447-455.

[35]   R. Marchioli, F. Barzi, E. Bomba *et al.* Early protection against sudden death by n-3 polyunsaturated fatty acids after myocardial infarction: time-course analysis of the results of the Gruppo Italiano per lo Studio della Sopravvivenza nell'Infarto Miocardico (GISSI)-Prevenzione. *Circulation* **105** (2002) 1897-1903.

[36]   R.B. Singh, M.A. Niaz, J.P. Sharma *et al.* Randomized, double-blind, placebo-controlled trial of fish oil and mustard oil in patients with suspected acute myocardial infarction: the Indian experiment of infarct survival-4. *Cardiovasc. Drugs Ther.* **11** (1997) 485-491.

[37]   C.M. Albert, H. Campos, M.J. Stampfer *et al.* Blood levels of long-chain n-3 fatty acids and the risk of sudden death. *N. Engl. J. Med.* **346** (2002) 1113-1118.

[38]   D. Mozaffarian, A. Ascherio, F.B. Hu *et al.* Interplay between different polyunsaturated fatty acids and risk of coronary heart disease in men. *Circulation* **111** (2005) 157-164.

[39]   K. He, Y. Song, M.L. Daviglus *et al.* Accumulated evidence on fish consumption and coronary heart disease mortality: a meta-analysis of cohort studies. *Circulation* **109** (2004) 2705-2711.

[40]   L. Djoussé, P.M. Rautaharju, P.N. Hopkins *et al.* Dietary linolenic acid and adjusted QT and JT intervals in the National Heart, Lung, and Blood Institute Family Heart study. *J. Am. Coll. Cardiol.* **45** (2005) 1716-1722.

[41]   A. Leaf, C.M. Albert, M. Josephson *et al.* Prevention of fatal arrhythmias on high-risk patients by fish oil n-3 fatty acid intake. *Circulation* **112** (2005) 2762-2768.

[42]   L. Calo, L. Bianconi, F. Colivicchi *et al.* N-3 fatty acids for the prevention of atrial fibrillation after coronary artery bypass surgery: a randomized, controlled trial. *J. Am. Coll. Cardiol.* **45** (2005) 1723-1728.

[43]   J.N. Din, D.E. Newby, A.D. Flapan. Omega 3 fatty acids and cardiovascular disease--fishing for a natural treatment. *BMJ* **328** (2004) 30-35.

[44]   F.B. Hu, L. Bronner, W.C. Willett *et al.* Fish and omega-3 fatty acid intake and risk of coronary heart disease in women. *JAMA* **287** (2002) 1815-1821.

[45]   K. Yoshizawa, E.B. Rimm, J.S. Morris *et al.* Mercury and the risk of coronary heart disease in men. *N. Engl. J. Med.* **347** (2002) 1755-1760.

[46]   E. Guallar, M.I. Sanz-Gallardo, P. van 't Veer *et al.* Mercury, fish oils and the risk of myocardial infarction. *N. Engl. J. Med.* **347** (2002) 1747-1754.

[47]   FDA. What you need to know about mercury in fish and shellfish. http://www.cfsan.fda.gov/~dms/admehg3b.html (2004).

[48]   C.N. Verboom, R. Marchioli, H. Rupp *et al.* Highly purified Omega-3 fatty acids for secondary prevention post-myocardial infarction. The Royal Society of Medicine Press Ltd. (2003). ISBN 1853155535.

[49]   H. Rupp, D. Wagner, T. Rupp *et al.* Risk stratification by the "EPA+DHA level" and the "EPA/AA ratio" focus on anti-inflammatory and antiarrhythmogenic effects of long-chain omega-3 fatty acids. *Herz* **29** (2004) 673-685.

[50]   R. Oh. Practical applications of fish oil (omega-3 fatty acids) in primary care. *J. Am. Board Fam. Pract.* **18** (2005) 28-36.

Omega-3 Fatty Acids and Sudden Arrhythmic Death

Stuart J. Connolly and Jeffrey S. Healey
Faculty of Health Sciences, McMaster University, 237 Barton Street E., Hamilton, Ontario L8L 2X2, Canada

Abstract. Prevention of Sudden Death after Acute Myocardial Infarction
Cardiovascular disease is the leading cause of death in developed countries. In Canada, in 1999, cardiovascular disease was responsible for 36% of all deaths. Ischemic heart disease accounts for the greatest percentage of these deaths (20% of all deaths), half of which are due to the acute effects of myocardial infarction. The other half are related to the late manifestations and complications of myocardial infarction [1]. Once coronary arteriosclerosis has reached the point where it results in myocardial infarction, two main complications can ensue, loss of myocardial function and disturbance of cardiac rhythm. Progressive loss of myocardial pump function results in the syndrome of congestive heart failure. Abnormalities of the heart rhythm result in ventricular fibrillation, which is the direct cause of sudden death. Congestive heart failure rates have been easy to track because of the frequent need for hospitalization and we know from analysis of administrative databases that the annual rate of death from heart failure is about 2.5% in Canada [1]. Sudden death, however most often occurs at home and without warning, making it much more difficult to quantitate its impact. However, the most conservative estimates suggest that no less than 25% of deaths in patients with a diagnosis of ischemic heart disease are due to ventricular fibrillation [2,3].

Keywords. Sudden death, cardiac arrhythmia, omega-3 fatty acid

Current Guidelines for Preventing Cardiovascular Complications after Myocardial Infarction

Major advances in the management and prevention of coronary disease and its complications have occurred in the past 30 years, lowering mortality rates from ischemic heart disease. Insights into the pathophysiology of atherosclerotic heart disease, development of effective pharmacological interventions and the use of clinical trials to prove their value have improved heart disease outcomes [4]. These advances have, as noted above, markedly lowered death rates from myocardial infarction, although total number of deaths has remained more or less constant due to the aging of the population. The use of antithrombotic and thrombolytic agents has mitigated the effects of acute coronary occlusion, lipid-lowering drugs slow the progression of atherosclerotic vascular disease. Renin-angiotensin system blockers reduce atherosclerosis and protect the myocardium. Beta-blockers reduce infarct size and slow progression of heart failure [5].

However when one considers that sudden arrhythmic death accounts for at least 25% of all cardiovascular death, it is striking that none of the agents currently recommended for post-myocardial infarction care has clear anti-arrhythmic activity. There currently are no anti-arrhythmic therapies available for survivors of myocardial infarction that can be routinely recommended [4].

Amiodarone has been extensively tested and is widely accepted to be a potent anti-arrhythmic agent. Results of large clinical trials in survivors of myocardial infarction, such as CAMIAT and EMIAT, have not shown a clear benefit of this agent [6].

Because of the significant toxicity associated with this drug and the lack of consistent reductions in mortality, amiodarone is not recommended routinely in survivors of myocardial infarction. Recently the Sudden Cardiac Death in Heart Failure Trial (SCDHFT) [2] convincingly showed that amiodarone does not reduce mortality in patients at high risk for sudden death.

Membrane active agents that reduce the risk of ventricular fibrillation in the animal laboratory have proved to be ineffective and even dangerous in patients [7]. The use of the implantable cardioverter defibrillator (ICD) reduces mortality in many high patients, but the recent results of the Defibrillators in Acute Myocardial Infarction Trial (DINAMIT) [3] clearly showed that in post-myocardial infarction patients the usual benefit seen with the ICD does not occur. This is likely due to the fact that the most common mechanism of arrhythmic death in these patients is ventricular fibrillation due to ischemia which is different from sustained ventricular tachycardia typically occurring in heart failure or in the very late phase (several years) after myocardial infarction. There is a need for well-tolerated safe therapies which reduce the risk of sudden death after recent myocardial infarction.

Omega-3 Fatty Acids

Omega-3 polyunsaturated fatty acids are of two types, α-linolenic acid that is derived from vegetable sources and two very long-chain polyunsaturated acids found in abundance in cold water marine life, eicosapentaenoic acid and docosahexaenoic acid (EPA and DHA). Omega-3 fatty acids modify biologic function in many ways [8]. Principally, they enter membrane phospholipids and alter membrane structure and function. Perhaps most importantly they modify the electrical activities of myocytes reducing the tendency for cardiac arrhythmia [9]. They can inhibit synthesis of pro-inflammatory cytokines and they reduce aggregational properties of blood platelets. They have a direct effect on triglyceride synthesis and lower triglyceride levels [10].

Epidemiological Evidence of Benefit

The evidence that omega-3 fatty acids are beneficial in the prevention of complications of cardiovascular disease first came from epidemiological observations. The early observations that Greenland Eskimos [11] suffered a low rate of cardiovascular death despite a diet exceeding high in fat (derived from marine mammals) lead to several major, within-population, prospective epidemiological studies which have shown that men and women who ate fish had a lower coronary heart disease mortality rate than those who ate none. In the Nurses Health Study [12], dietary consumption of fish and follow-up clinical outcome data from validated questionnaires performed over a 14-year period were compared from 84,688 female nurses, aged 34-59 years.

The purpose of the study was to examine the relationship between fish and omega-3 fatty acid consumption and the risk of coronary artery disease. As can be seen in Table 1, there was a strong inverse relationship between fish consumption and coronary heart disease events, even after adjustment for multiple co-variates such as age, body-mass index, smoking, etc.

Table 1. Fish consumption and coronary heart disease (CHD) events in the Nurses Health Study [12]

Fish consumption frequency	Relative risk of CHD	95% confidence interval
<1 per month	1	
1-3 per month	0.79	0.64-0.97
1 per week	0.71	0.58-0.87
2-4 per week	0.69	0.55-0.88

In the thirty-year follow-up of the Chicago Western Electric study, men who consumed high quantities of fish had almost a 40% lower risk of death from coronary heart disease than men who consumed no fish at all [13]. The US Physicians' Health Study reported a 52% decrease in sudden cardiac death in subjects who ate fish at least once per week [14]. There was no decrease in myocardial infarction, and no incremental benefit seen with greater fish consumption. In the Zutphen study, Kromhout *et al* showed that mortality from coronary heart disease was more than 50% lower among those who consumed at least 30 gm of fish per day than among those who did not eat fish [15].

A recent meta-analysis [16] of epidemiological studies was performed to examine the relationship between fish intake and coronary heart mortality. This analysis included data from over 200,000 individuals with an average follow-up of 11.8 years. Compared to people who never ate fish or ate it less than once per month, this study reported significant reduced relative risk for coronary mortality that was strongly related to fish intake. The relative risks for coronary mortality were 0.89 for fish intake of 1-3 times per month, 0.77 for fish intake of 2-4 times per week and 0.62 for fish intake of 5 or more times per week. Each 20 gm per day increase in fish intake resulted in a 7% lower risk of coronary heart disease mortality (p=0.03). Figure 1 shows the meta-analysis results.

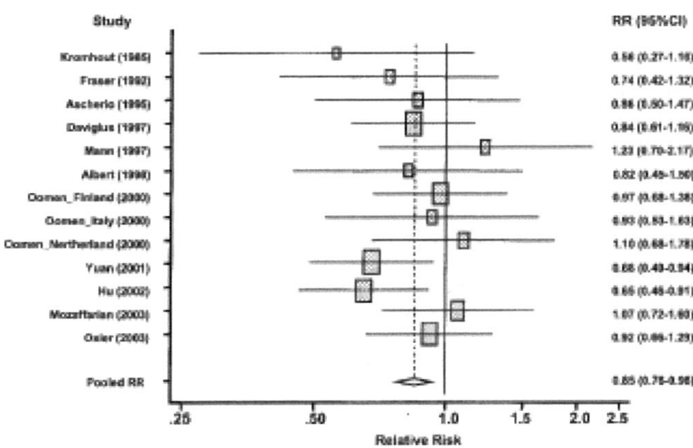

Figure 1. Pooled estimate of RR and 95% CI of CHD mortality rates for fish consumption 1/week vs. <1/month. Squares indicate adjusted RR in each study. Size of the square is proportional to the percent weight of each study in the meta-analysis; horizontal line represents 95% CI. Studies are ordered by year of publication. Pooled RR and 95% CI are indicated by the unshaded diamond.

In conclusion, most epidemiological studies have supported a clear association between the fish intake and reduced mortality from cardiovascular disease, and the overwhelming consensus of experts is that a strong association between dietary intake of omega-3 fatty acids and reduced coronary mortality exists [8].

Clinical Trials of Omega-3 Fatty Acids

Extensive epidemiological evidence that omega-3 fatty acids were protective against cardiovascular disease outcomes led to the organization of randomized controlled trials, several of which have been supportive and one of which was a definitive landmark study.

The first of these was the Diet And Reinfarction Trial (DART), reported in 1989 [17]. In this trial 2,033 male survivors of acute myocardial infarction (mean of 41 days post-MI) were randomized to receive or not receive advice on 3 different dietary interventions (a factorial 2x2x2 design). The interventions were a) to increase fatty fish intake to >1 fish meal per week, b) to lower fat intake and c) to increase fibre intake.

Subjects intolerant of fish took concentrated fish oil capsules. This trial reported a statistically significant 29% reduction in all-cause mortality in those who were advised to increase fish intake, during a two-year follow-up. The greatest benefit was seen in fatal recurrence of myocardial infarction, which suggested that the omega-3 fatty acids might be reducing the risk of fatal arrhythmia associated with acute myocardial infarction. More recently, Singh *et al* [18] reported the results of a trial performed in patients admitted to hospital with suspected acute MI. Patients were randomized three ways, a) to fish oil capsules containing 1.8 gm per day of EPA and DHA, b) to capsules containing mustard oil high in α-linolenic acid, or c) to placebo. After one year of follow-up, total cardiac events were significantly less with the use of capsules containing the omega-3 fatty acids, EPA and DHA compared with the placebo group (25% vs. 35%; p<0.01).

GISSI-Prevention Study

The epidemiological data and the results of DART led to the organization of the GISSI-Prevention trial [19] which was designed to provide definitive evidence regarding the benefit of omega-3 fatty acid supplementation for the prevention of vascular events during the late follow-up after acute myocardial infarction. Between October 1993 to September 1995, 11,324 patients surviving recent ($\leq$3 months) myocardial infarction were randomly assigned to receive once daily supplements of the highly concentrated, purified, omega-3 fatty acid preparation or to control.

This preparation contained 1 gm of EPA and DHA. GISSI-Prevention was a two-way factorial designed trial and thus patients were also separately randomized to receive a daily supplement of 300 mg of vitamin E or to control. Mean follow-up was 3.5 years. The primary combined efficacy end-points of the trial were: 1) the cumulative rate of all-cause death, non-fatal myocardial infarction and non-fatal stroke; 2) the cumulative rate of cardiovascular death, non-fatal myocardial infarction and non-fatal stroke.

Study medications were administered over and above all of the standard medications used in the management of survivors of acute myocardial infarction. A snapshot of concomitant medications at 42 months after randomization showed that 83% of patients were receiving an anti-platelet drug, 39% were receiving an angiotensin-converting enzyme inhibitor, 39% were receiving a beta-blocker, 46% were receiving cholesterol-lowering drugs. In addition, 24% of patients in the study received a coronary revascularization procedure during the course of the study. Dietary habits at baseline and during the study were well-balanced across all groups. More than 73% of patients had at least 1 fish meal served per week, 80% ate fruit and 40% ate fresh vegetables at least once a day, and more than 73% used olive oil regularly. The median time from admission to hospital for acute myocardial infarction until randomization was 16 days. Patients randomized to receive omega-3 fatty acids were well-matched in regard to major prognostic factors with patients randomized to control.

The primary study result was a 15% decrease (p=0.023) in the relative risk of the combined primary end-point (the composite of death, non-fatal myocardial infarction and non-fatal stroke) with omega-3 fatty acids compared to control. An analysis of the individual components of the main end-point showed that omega-3 fatty capsules resulted in statistically significant reductions of 20% in total deaths, of 30% in cardiovascular deaths and of 45% in sudden death. However, omega-3 fatty acids did not reduce non-fatal infarction. This pattern of effects suggests that the predominant mechanism of action of omega-3 fatty acids in infarction survivors is to stabilize the heart rhythm.

In the other primary analysis of GISSI-Prevention, patients randomized to receive vitamin E or to control did not differ significantly in the primary outcome or any of its components, when data were analyzed according to the factorial design. The once daily dose of omega-3 fatty acids was well-tolerated. Side-effects were uncommon and included gastrointestinal disturbance and nausea. Only 3.8% of patients receiving omega-3 fatty acids discontinued because of side-effects.

GISSI-Prevention and Reduction in Sudden Death

The striking and large reduction in sudden death prompted the GISSI-Prevention investigators to provide further analysis of their data [20], which is contained in a recent report that examines the time-course of the mortality reduction and cause specific mortality. Analysis of the time-course of the appearance of the effects of omega-3 fatty acid supplementation showed an early and highly significant reduction in sudden cardiac death, which is the major component of the total mortality reduction. Conversely, there was no indication of a decrease in non-fatal myocardial infarction.

These results suggest that anti-arrhythmic and anti-fibrillatory effects of omega-3 fatty acids are very important components in the mortality benefit. Patients allocated to omega-3 fatty acids had significantly lower mortality even after only three months of treatment (1.1% vs. 1.6%); relative risk 0.59, (p=0.037). The reduction in sudden death was nearly statistically significant after only three months of treatment and it accounted for 57% of the overall mortality benefit at that time. The sudden death mortality reduction became significant at four months and was highly significant at 42 months (2.0% vs. 2.7%); relative risk 0.55, (p=0.0006). At the end of the study it accounted for 59% of the omega-3 fatty acid advantage on mortality. Figure 2 shows the time-course of treatment effects for various components of the reduction in total mortality from the GISSI-Prevention trial.

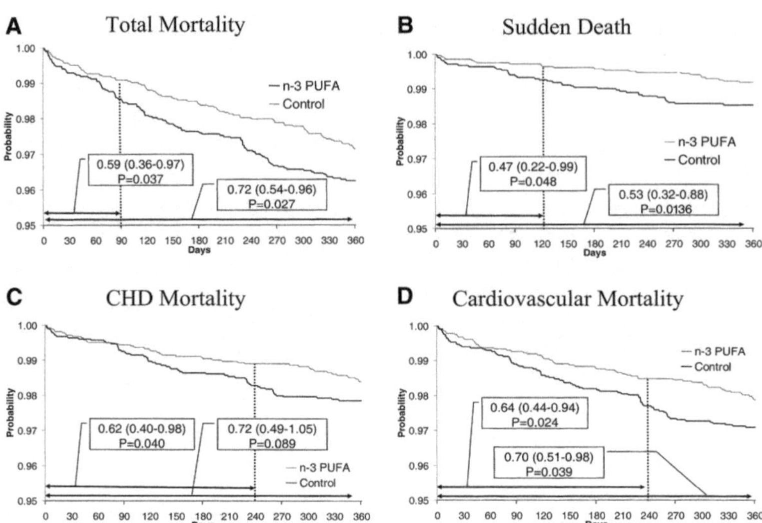

Figure 2. Fatal outcomes from GISSI-Prevention [20].

These analyses indicate that omega-3 fatty acids reduce total mortality after myocardial infarction in large part by reducing sudden death and they strongly suggest that there is a direct anti-arrhythmic action.

Omega-3 Fatty Acids and Sudden Death

There is considerable basic experimental evidence that supports a direct anti-arrhythmic action for omega-3 fatty acids. In '*in vitro*' studies with cultured neonatal rat myocytes, DHA and EPA have been shown to modify voltage-dependent activation of sodium channels such that the size of the electrical stimulus required to depolarize the cell is increased by 50%, an effect that could increase electrical stability [9]. The omega-3 fatty acids have also been show to affect the L-type calcium current to prevent excessive influx of calcium into the cell, protecting the cell from calcium overload [9]. EPA has been shown to be protective against the effects of increased calcium and ouabain on the spontaneously beating cultured neonatal rat myocytes by preventing the induction of rapid contractions, contractures, and fibrillation of the myocytes [21,22].

In a feeding study of rats, it has been reported that the rate of ventricular fibrillation after coronary ligation is significantly reduced if rats are fed a diet high in omega-3 fatty acids compared to diets either high in saturated fatty acids or high in olive oil [23]. The rates of ventricular fibrillation with the saturated fat diet compared to with the omega-3 fatty acid diet were 40% and 0%, respectively. Billman *et al* [24] have shown that intravenous administration of EPA or DHA reduced ventricular fibrillation in a well-characterized dog model of ischemic sudden death. This model of sudden cardiac death has been developed using a surgically induced anterior myocardial infarction and a hydraulic, inflatable cuff around the left circumflex coronary artery that can be compressed at will. The dogs are trained to run on a treadmill and are recovered from the surgery and the anterior myocardial infarction. With exercise and occlusion of the left circumflex artery, most of the dogs go into a fatal ventricular fibrillation within 2 minutes of the compression of the artery. In this model omega-3 fatty infusion just before exercise, reduced the risk of ventricular fibrillation. Infusions of both linolenic acid, EPA and DHA were also effective. Results are shown in Table 2.

Table 2. Prevention of ischemia-induced fatal ventricular arrhythmias by n-3 polyunsaturated fatty acids in a dog model of sudden cardiac death

| | No. of Dogs Tested | | |
n-3 PUFAs	Total	Protected	P
Fish oil concentrate*	13	10	<0.005
EPA†	7	5	<0.02
DHA††	8	6	<0.004
α-LNA§	8	6	<0.004

*72% n-3 PUFA with free EPA 33.9% and DHA 25%.
†98.4% free EPA; 1.1% free DHA.
††90.8% free DHA; 0.9% free EPA.
§>99% free ALA.

Until recently there has been little research done in humans to examine the anti-arrhythmic effects of omega-3 fatty acids. Reduced heart rate variability in survivors of myocardial infarction is associated with an increased risk of sudden death. In one study, consumption of omega-3 fatty acid supplements increased heart rate variability in myocardial infarction survivors [25]. In another study of 7 patients with implantable defibrillators [26], infusion of omega-3 fatty acid was performed before electrophysiological study. Fatty acid infusion induced a significant prolongation of the effective refractory period of the right ventricle. In 5 of 7 patients with inducible sustained ventricular tachycardia immediately before infusion, sustained tachycardia could not be induced after infusion of the omega-3 fatty acids.

A recent study [27] has evaluated omega-3 fatty acid treatment in patients undergoing coronary artery bypass surgery to determine the effect of this agent on the occurrence of postoperative atrial fibrillation. A total of 160 patients were prospectively randomized to a control group (81 patients, 13 female, mean age 64.9 years) or to omega-3 fatty acid treatment 2 g/day (79 patients, 11 female, mean age 66.2 years) for at least 5 days before elective CABG and until the day of discharge from the hospital. Postoperative atrial fibrillation developed in 27 patients of the control group (33.3%) and in 12 patients of the fatty acid group (15.2%) (p=0.013). This is the first study to show that omega-3 fatty acids have an anti-fibrillatory effect in the atrium.

A small trial of omega-3 fatty acids has been done in patients with implantable cardioverter defibrillators (ICDs) to determine whether omega-3 fatty acids have anti-arrhythmic effects in patients with a history of sustained ventricular tachycardia or ventricular fibrillation (VT/VF) [28]. A randomized, double-blind, placebo-controlled trial was performed at 6 US medical centers with enrollment of 200 patients all of whom had an ICD and a recent episode of sustained VT or VF. They were randomly assigned to receive fish oil, 1.8 g/d, (72% omega-3 fatty acids) or placebo, and were followed up for a median of 718 days. The primary outcome was time to first episode of ICD treatment for VT/VF. Patients randomized to receive fish oil had an increase in the mean percentage of omega-3 fatty acids in red blood cell membranes from 4.7% to 8.3% (p<0.001), with no change observed in patients receiving placebo. At 6, 12, and 24 months, 46%, 51% and 65% of patients randomized to receive omega-3 fatty acids had ICD therapy for VT/VF compared with 36%, 41% and 59% for patients randomized to receive placebo (p=0.19).

Recurrent VT/VF events were more common in patients randomized to receive fish oil (p<0.001). The authors concluded that among patients with a recent episode of sustained ventricular arrhythmia and an ICD, fish oil supplementation does not reduce the risk of VT/VF.

This very small study does not confirm that omega-3 fatty acids are anti-arrhythmic, however the study was clearly too small to be definitive. A somewhat larger ICD study is now underway in Europe that will provide some useful data. It is worth noting that ICD patients are very different from survivors of recent myocardial infarction who were studied in the GISSI-Prevention trial. ICD patients typically have monomorphic ventricular tachycardia which is often not fatal and which has a different mechanism from the arrhythmias that may occur in the early months after myocardial infarction where recurrent ischemic events are more common. The results of DINAMIT trial [3] have recently drawn attention to the differences between chronic ventricular arrhythmias which respond well to an ICD and the arrhythmias that occur early after myocardial infarction that do not respond to the ICD. In summary, *in vitro* and *in vivo* studies show that omega-3 fatty acids have direct effects on ventricular arrhythmias, but in man direct anti-arrhythmic activity has not been demonstrated. Further studies are needed to better define the anti-arrhythmic activity of omega-3 fatty acids in patients.

Other studies have suggested potential other mechanisms to explain the reduction in sudden death seen in the GISSI-Prevention trial, such as increased stability of atherosclerotic plaque. A placebo-controlled randomized treatment study of patients awaiting carotid endarterectomy reported that patients randomized pre-surgery to treatment with concentrated omega-3 fatty supplementation showed clear incorporation of EPA and DHA into diseased carotid plaque, less evidence of inflammation and thicker fibrous caps [29]. If omega-3 fatty acids produce similar effects in the coronary artery (which is likely) this would explain a lower risk of acute plaque rupture, which can cause sudden death.

Dietary Fish Intake and Mercury Contamination

Expert opinion in the dietary field now favors moderate increases in the dietary intakes of plant-derived α-linolenic acid based upon the epidemiologic evidence of reduction in cardiovascular outcomes [8]. Recommendations regarding increased dietary intake of fish have been modulated by concern about the risk of increased exposure to mercury. Mercury is a highly reactive heavy metal which is toxic at all doses. The long-term consequences of exposure to, even low, levels of mercury are poorly understood [8]. Fish intake is a major source of human exposure to mercury.

A recent study showed that increased concentration of mercury in human nail clippings was associated with a risk of increased cardiovascular events [30]. When adipose concentrations of DHA were also accounted for in that analysis, the data suggested that the beneficial effects of the omega-3 fatty acid, DHA, on cardiovascular outcomes were offset by detrimental effects of mercury.

Cardiology Society Guideline Recommendations

A wealth of epidemiological data supports a protective role for omega-3 fatty acids against cardiovascular outcomes. A very large, well-performed, major randomized trial provides strong evidence that a once daily dose of a concentrated, mercury free, preparation of omega-3 fatty acid containing 1 gm of EPA and DHA reduces cardiovascular outcomes in survivors of myocardial infarction [18]. There is good evidence that a major mechanism of benefit of omega-3 fatty acids is prevention of sudden death. Several other studies support the direct anti-arrhythmic mechanism of omega-3 fatty acids. An American Heart Association Scientific statement [8] indicates that physicians should consider supplements of omega-3 fatty acids for patients with coronary artery disease for coronary heart disease risk reduction. The 2002 European Society of Cardiology task force report [31] on the management of myocardial infarction specifically recommends (Class 1, level of evidence B) supplementation with 1 gm fish oil n-3 polyunsaturated fatty acids for the long-term management of survivors of myocardial infarction [24].

References

[1]   Heart and Stroke Foundation of Canada. The growing burden of heart disease and stroke in Canada 2003. Ottawa, Canada (2003).

[2]   G.H. Bardy, K.L. Lee, D.B. Mark *et al.* Sudden Cardiac Death in Heart Failure Trial (SCD-HeFT) Investigators. Amiodarone or an implantable cardioverter-defibrillator for congestive heart failure. *N. Engl. J. Med.* **352** (2005) 225-237.

[3]   S.H. Hohnloser, K.H. Kuck, P. Dorian *et al.* DINAMIT Investigators. Prophylactic use of an implantable cardioverter-defibrillator after acute myocardial infarction. *N. Engl. J. Med.* **351** (2004) 2481-2488.

[4]   S.C. Smith Jr, S.N. Blair, R.O. Bonow *et al.* AHA/ACC Scientific Statement: AHA/ACC guidelines for preventing heart attack and death in patients with atherosclerotic cardiovascular disease: 2001 update: A statement for healthcare professionals from the American Heart Association and the American College of Cardiology. *Circulation* **104** (2001) 1577-1579.

[5]   M. Gheorghiade and S. Goldstein. Beta-blockers in the post-myocardial infarction patient. *Circulation* **106** (2002) 394-398.

[6]   S.M. Jafri, S. Borzak, J. Goldberger *et al.* Role of antiarrhythmic agents after myocardial infarction with special reference to the EMIAT and CAMIAT trials of amiodarone. European Myocardial Infarct Amiodarone Trial. Canadian Amiodarone Myocardial Infarction Trial. *Prog. Cardiovasc. Dis.* **41** (1998) 65-70.

[7]   J.A. Larsen, A.H. Kadish, J.B. Schwartz. Proper use of antiarrhythmic therapy for reduction of mortality after myocardial infarction. *Drugs Aging* **16** (2000) 341-350.

[8]   P.M. Kris-Etherton, W.S. Harris, L.J. Appel. Fish consumption, fish oil, omega-3 fatty acids, and cardiovascular disease. *Circulation* **106** (2002) 2747-2757.

[9]   Y.F. Xiao, D.C. Sigg, A. Leaf. The antiarrhythmic effect of n-3 polyunsaturated fatty acids: modulation of cardiac ion channels as a potential mechanism. *J. Membr. Biol.* **206** (2005) 141-154.

[10]   H.C. Hsu, Y.T. Lee, M.F. Chen. Effect of n-3 fatty acids on the composition and binding properties of lipoproteins in hypertriglyceridemic patients. *Am. J. Clin. Nutr.* **71** (2000) 28-35.

[11]   H.O. Bang, J. Dyerberg, H.M. Sinclair. The composition of the Eskimo food in north western Greenland. *Am. J. Clin. Nutr.* **33** (1980) 2657-2661.

[12]   F.B. Hu, L. Bronner, W.C. Willett *et al.* Fish and omega-3 fatty acid intake and risk of coronary heart disease in women. *JAMA* **287** (2002) 1815-1821.

[13]   M.L. Daviglus, J. Stamler, A.J. Orencia *et al.* Fish consumption and the 30-year risk of fatal myocardial infarction. *N. Engl. J. Med.* **336** (1997) 1046-1053.

[14]   C.M. Albert, C.H. Hennekens, C.J. O'Donnell *et al.* Fish consumption and risk of sudden cardiac death. *JAMA* **279** (1998) 23-28.

[15]   D. Kromhout, E.B. Bosschieter, C. de Lezenne Coulander. The inverse relation between fish consumption and 20-year mortality from coronary heart disease. *N. Engl. J. Med.* **312** (1985) 1205-1209.

[16]   K. He, Y. Song, M.L. Daviglus *et al.* Accumulated evidence on fish consumption and coronary heart disease mortality: a meta-analysis of cohort studies. *Circulation* **109** (2004) 2705-2711.

[17]   M.L. Burr, A.M. Fehily, J.F. Gilbert *et al.* Effects of changes in fat, fish, and fibre intakes on death and myocardial reinfarction: diet and reinfarction trial (DART). *Lancet* **2** (1989) 757-761.

[18]   R.B. Singh, M.A. Niaz, J.P. Sharma *et al.* Randomized, double-blind, placebo-controlled trial of fish oil and mustard oil in patients with suspected acute myocardial infarction: the Indian experiment of infarct survival - 4. *Cardiovasc. Drugs Ther.* **11** (1997) 485-491.

[19]   GISSI-Prevenzione Investigators. Dietary supplementation with n-3 polyunsaturated fatty acids and vitamin E after myocardial infarction: results of the GISSI-Prevenzione trial. Gruppo Italiano per lo Studio della Sopravvivenza nell'Infarto Miocardico. *Lancet* **354** (1999) 447-455.

[20]   R. Marchioli, F. Barzi, E. Bomba *et al.* Early protection against sudden death by n-3 polyunsaturated fatty acids after myocardial infarction: time-course analysis of the results of the Gruppo Italiano per lo Studio della Sopravvivenza nell'Infarto Miocardico (GISSI)-Prevenzione. *Circulation* **105** (2002) 1897-1903.

[21]   J.X. Kang and A. Leaf. Effects of long-chain polyunsaturated fatty acids on the contraction of neonatal rat cardiac myocytes. *Proc. Natl. Acad. Sci. U.S.A.* **91** (1994) 9886-9890.

[22]   J.X. Kang and A. Leaf. Prevention and termination effect of beta-adrenergic agonist-induced arrhythmias by free polyunsaturated fatty acids in neonatal rat cardiac myocytes. *Biochem. Biophys. Res. Comm.* **208** (1995) 629-636

[23]   P.L. McLennan. Relative effects of dietary saturated, monounsaturated, and polyunsaturated fatty acids on cardiac arrhythmias in rats. *Am. J. Clin. Nutr.* **57** (1993) 207-212.

[24]   G.E. Billman, J.X. Kang, A. Leaf. Prevention of sudden cardiac death by dietary pure omega-3 polyunsaturated fatty acids in dogs. *Circulation* **99** (1999) 2452-2457.

[25]   J.H. Christensen, E. Korup, J. Aaroe *et al.* Fish consumption, n-3 fatty acids in cell membranes, and heart rate variability in survivors of myocardial infarction with left ventricular dysfunction. *Am. J. Cardiol.* **79** (1997) 1670-1673.

[26]   R. Schrepf, T. Limmert, P.C. Weber *et al.* Immediate effects of n-3 fatty acid infusion on the induction of sustained ventricular tachycardia. *Lancet* **363** (2004) 1441-1442.

[27]   M.H. Raitt, W.E. Connor, C. Morris *et al.* Fish oil supplementation and risk of ventricular tachycardia and ventricular fibrillation in patients with implantable defibrillators: a randomized controlled trial. *JAMA* **293** (2005) 2884-2891.

[28]   L. Calo, L. Bianconi, F. Colivicchi *et al.* N-3 fatty acids for the prevention of atrial fibrillation after coronary artery bypass surgery: a randomized, controlled trial. *J. Am. Coll. Cardiol.* **45** (2005) 1723-1728.

[29]   F. Thies, J.M. Garry, P. Yaqoob *et al.* Association of n-3 polyunsaturated fatty acids with stability of atherosclerotic plaques: a randomised controlled trial. *Lancet* **361** (2003) 477-485.

[30]   E. Guallar, M.I. Sanz-Gallardo, P. van 't Veer *et al.* Mercury, fish oils, and the risk of myocardial infarction. *N. Engl. J. Med.* **347** (2002) 1747-1754.

[31]   F. van de Werf, D. Ardissino, A. Betriu *et al.* Management of acute myocardial infarction in patients presenting with ST-segment elevation. The Task Force on the Management of Acute Myocardial Infarction of the European Society of Cardiology. *Eur. Heart J.* **24** (2003) 28-66.

Cardiovascular Benefits of Omega-3 Polyunsaturated Fatty Acids
B. Maisch and R. Oelze (Eds.)
IOS Press, 2006

Depression and Coronary Artery Disease: Epidemiology and Potential Mechanisms

Nancy Frasure-Smith and François Lespérance
*Centre Hospitalier de l'Université de Montréal, Hôpital Notre-Dame, Recherche
Psychiatrie, Pavillon L-C Simard, 1560 rue Sherbrooke Est, Montréal, Québec,
Canada H2L 4M1*

Abstract. Studies in patients recovering from myocardial infarction, episodes of unstable angina, coronary bypass surgery and coronary angioplasty, show that between 12 and 20% of hospitalized cardiac patients meet psychiatric criteria for current major depression. A similar percentage report elevated levels of depressive symptoms on paper and pencil self-report measures. These rates of depression are about three times higher than in the general community. On a practical basis this means that about one in three hospitalized CAD patients has some degree of depression. Despite its high prevalence in patients with CAD, depression is not a normal reaction to cardiac disease. Both major depression and elevated depressive symptoms are associated with at least a doubling in risk of subsequent cardiac events, even when standard cardiac risk factors, including left ventricular ejection fraction and number of blocked coronary arteries, are taken into account. In fact, several large, longitudinal community-based studies show that depression precedes the development of clinically evident CAD by many years. There is substantial evidence that depression is a potentially modifiable cardiac risk factor of as much importance as diabetes or lack of exercise. Although the precise mechanisms explaining the link between depression and CAD remain unknown, there is evidence that changes in autonomic regulation, sub-chronic inflammation, endothelial dysfunction, enhanced platelet responsiveness and reduced omega-3 free fatty acid levels may all be involved. Intriguingly, the mechanisms that have been hypothesized to explain the link between depression and CAD prognosis are the same as those suggested to explain the favorable impact of omega-3 supplements in CAD patients. Additional clinical trials to assess the impact of omega-3 supplements on depression are clearly warranted both in CAD patients and in individuals free of heart disease.

Keywords. Depression, CAD, prognosis, omega-3

Introduction

In 1997 the Global Burden of Disease Study concluded that in industrialized nations coronary artery disease (CAD) is the leading cause of early death and disability [1]. This was not surprising to most clinicians and researchers working in the cardiovascular field. What was surprising, was that the second leading cause was depression, and that both depression and CAD are increasing in prevalence around the world. In fact, the authors went on to forecast that by the year 2020 CAD and depression would be the two leading causes of death and disability on a worldwide basis. In the context of the increasing evidence of epidemiological and physiological links between depression and CAD, which are summarized in the following paragraphs, research into treatments that may target both conditions is of high importance. The evidence of the pleiotropic effects of omega-3 fatty acids on many of the systems involved in depression and CAD makes omega-3 supplementation an important candidate for trials of depression treatment and prevention.

Definitions and Prevalence

In clinical terms, depression is not just having the blues or feeling down for a couple of days. Although sadness and lack of interest are the cardinal symptoms of depression, several other symptoms are usually present. In addition, people who are depressed have enough difficulty functioning normally in their day to day lives to justify treatment. According to the Diagnostic and Statistical Manual (version IV) of the American Psychiatric Association [2], to be considered as having major depression, an individual must have experienced sadness or loss of interest plus enough of the following symptoms to have a total of at least five symptoms: changes in appetite, changes in sleep patterns, psychomotor agitation or retardation, loss of energy or fatigue, feelings of worthlessness, inability to concentrate or make decisions, and thoughts of suicide or death. Further, these symptoms have to have been present on an almost daily basis for at least two weeks and resulted in impairment in fulfilling normal roles. Although studies have varied in the time period used to define major depression, prevalence estimates in hospitalized cardiac patients, including post-myocardial infarction (MI) [3], unstable angina [4], congestive heart failure [5], post-bypass [6] and angiography [7], consistently show that at least 14 to 20 percent are depressed. There is another group at least as large, who have a combination of various depression symptoms, but who do not meet DSM-IV criteria for major depression. In fact, when measured with self-report, pen and pencil type instruments, at least one in three hospitalized cardiac patients shows some degree of depressive symptomatology [8]. Although comparable to the prevalence of depression in other groups with chronic medical conditions [9], depression is about three times as common in CAD patients as in the general community [10].

Prognosis in Established CAD

Depression is common in cardiac patients, but this does not mean that it is normal. As for depression in general [11], in CAD patients depression is a chronic and debilitating disease. For example, we followed 220 post-MI patients with depression evaluations in hospital for one year, and found that among those with no evidence of depression at baseline, 86% were alive and depression-free at the time of the one-year follow-up [12]. This was in stark contrast to only 31% of those with major depression during hospitalization, and 52% of those with elevated depression symptoms who did not meet psychiatric criteria for major depression.

Even more striking than the chronicity of untreated depression in cardiac patients, is the evidence of its links with prognosis. We recently reviewed the literature on depression and CAD published before 2004 [13]. When we took multiple publications from the same database into account (for example, different follow-up periods for the same sample), we found 30 studies with samples of more than 100 patients that had prospective designs, used recognized measures of depression and had objective cardiac outcomes. The majority (19) showed depression to be a significant predictor of prognosis even after adjustment for measures of cardiac disease severity. However, according to our calculations "assuming a 30% prevalence for elevated depressive symptoms and an overall 1-year mortality of 10%, a sample of more than 600 would be needed to have at least 80% power (two-tailed alpha = 0.05) to detect a doubling in risk associated with depressive symptoms" [13]. Only one of the studies that did not find a significant relationship between depression and prognosis had this large a sample. That study involved one of the first measures of depression ever developed that is no longer in use today, and a later publication from the same database using a revised measure and a longer follow-up, did observe a significant link between depression and prognosis. In fact, a recent meta-analysis of the impact of elevated depression symptoms during hospitalization on mortality from 3 months to two years after the event, reported a combined odds ratio for mortality associated with depression of 2.24 (95% confidence interval 1.39-3.60) [14].

There is also evidence of a dose-response relationship between levels of depression symptoms and prognosis. We assessed depression symptoms in a hospitalized sample of 896 post-MI patients receiving usual care from their physicians, and followed them for five years [15]. The higher the number of depression symptoms the greater the long-term risk. Further, this dose-response relationship remained significant after adjustment for measures of cardiac disease severity, with the level of increased risk comparable to that observed with standard risks like previous MI and diabetes. Even more striking was the fact that the dose-response pattern was equally apparent when we analyzed the cognitive symptoms (sadness, loss of interest, inability to concentrate etc.) and the somatic symptoms of depression (fatigue, appetite, sleep etc.) separately (see Figure 1).

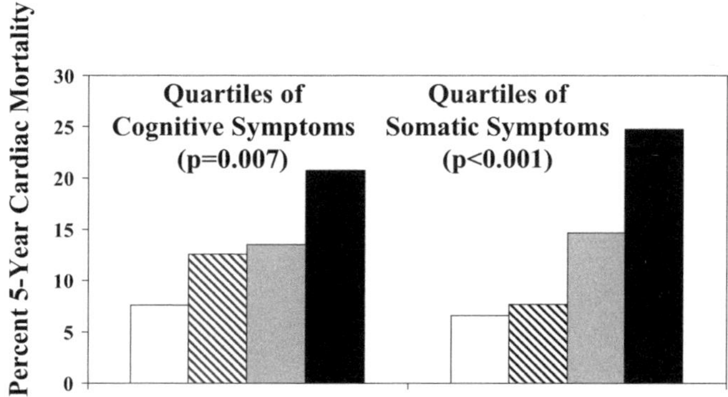

Figure 1. Long-term survival impact of increasing levels of cognitive and somatic symptoms of depression after myocardial infarction (BDI, n = 896).

Depression as a Risk Factor for the Development of CAD

Although there have not been as many studies of the etiological importance of depression for the development of CAD, the results of those that have been published are remarkably consistent. In our review of the literature prior to 2004 [13] discussed previously, we identified 15 independent studies of CAD incidence that used recognized measures of depression, samples of more than 500 individuals and longitudinal designs. Eleven of these found significant associations between depression and the development of CAD. Limiting the outcome to all-cause mortality, seven of eight studies showed a significant relationship. In fact, a meta-analysis of 11 cohort studies published prior to 2000, that measured depressive mood or major depression and evaluated incident MI or cardiac disease was carried out by Rugulies *et al* [16]. Overall they observed an increased relative risk of CAD of 1.64 (95% confidence interval 1.29-2.08, p<0.001) associated with either depressive mood or major depression.

Recently, two other important studies examining depression as a risk factor for incident CAD were published. The results of the Women's Health Initiative (WHI) study [17], that followed more than 70,000 postmenopausal women without a history of cardiovascular disease over four years, showed that elevated depression symptoms at baseline significantly predicted cardiovascular death even after adjustment for age, race, education, income and cardiac risk factors (adjusted relative risk = 1.50, 95% confidence interval = 1.10 - 2.03). The second recent study is INTERHEART [18], a case-control study of more than 11,000 first MI cases and age and sex matched controls in 52 countries. INTERHEART reported a population attributable risk (PAR) of about 9% associated with depression in the year previous to the MI. This was independent of age, sex, region and current smoking status, and comparable to the PAR for MI associated with diabetes (9.9%). The PAR takes into account the prevalence of the risk factor and the size of its link to outcome, and suggests that if depression (or diabetes) were completely eliminated there would be about 9% fewer first MIs per year on a worldwide basis.

Summary of Epidemiological Studies of Depression and CAD

Whether depression is assessed with self-report measures of depressive symptoms or psychiatric interviews to establish criteria for a current episode of major depression, depression is common in CAD patients. Most depression is more than a short-term reaction to the stresses of experiencing a cardiac event. Studies have consistently showed the depressed to be at significantly increased risk of cardiac mortality and readmissions to hospital. The increase in risk associated with depression is about the same as that associated with standard risk factors like previous MI and diabetes, and statistically independent of measures of cardiac disease severity.

Mechanisms

While the mechanisms linking depression and CAD remain unknown, many potential pathways have been suggested, including behavioral, pathophysiologic and genetic mechanisms [19,20]. There is evidence that depressed patients are less likely to adhere to recommendations for risk factor modification [21], and to take medications as prescribed [22]. One study has suggested that patients with affective disorders (the combination of anxiety disorders and mood disorders) may be less likely to undergo cardiac catheterization [23], so there may be depression-related differences in the timing and type of cardiac treatment received. Beyond this, depression is associated with autonomic dysregulation (including reduced heart rate variability (HRV) and increased risk of ventricular arrhythmias) [3,24], markers of inflammation [25,26], endothelial dysfunction [27,28] and changes in platelet activation [29,30], many of which have themselves been linked to cardiac prognosis in other research.

Omega-3 fatty acid levels may also play a role. Several epidemiological studies have demonstrated lower levels of long-chain polyunsaturated fatty acids (PUFAs) in depressed individuals in comparison to the non-depressed in samples without CAD [31-34]. We recently confirmed these findings in stable CAD patients assessed approximately two months after an admission for acute coronary syndrome [35]. Our case-control study of PUFA levels involved 54 CAD patients with current major depression and 54 age- and sex-matched CAD controls. The depressed had significantly lower concentrations of docosahexaenoic acid (DHA) and total omega-3, and higher ratios of arachidonic acid (AA) to eicosapentaenoic acid (EPA), AA to DHA, and total omega-6 to omega-3 levels than the non-depressed.

To date few studies have prospectively measured depression, potential mechanisms and cardiac events in order to assess the importance of different pathophysiological pathways in explaining the association between depression and CAD. One of the few was recently published by Carney and colleagues [36]. They followed a group of 358 depressed post-MI patients and a control group of 408 who were depression-free at baseline for 30 months. As in the studies published prior to 2004, summarized earlier, the authors found depression to be significantly linked to cardiac mortality (hazards ratio = 3.1, 95% confidence interval = 1.6 to 5.9, p<0.001). Cross-sectional results of the relationship between depression at baseline and spectral analysis of 24-hour HRV showed the depressed to have significantly lower ultra-low, very low, and low frequency HRV indices [24]. However, the prospective follow-up showed that only 27% of depression's link to cardiac mortality was explained by HRV. Further, multivariate analysis showed that depression, HRV and a composite measure of cardiac risk had statistically significant impacts on cardiac mortality that were largely independent of each other. Thus, while decreased HRV, and greater cardiac disease severity are two pathways linking depression and cardiac prognosis, they are not the complete story. Some other mechanism(s) is/are likely to be involved.

Although not yet evaluated in patients with established CAD, a nested, case-control study included in the Prospective Epidemiological Study of Myocardial Infarction (PRIME) examined the importance of several inflammatory markers as mediators of the relationship between depression and cardiac events in initially healthy men [37]. The results, involving 304 cases with incident cardiac events over a five- to six-year period and 585 controls, showed that depressive mood was significantly related to cardiac events (odds ratio = 1.35, 95% confidence interval 1.05 to 1.73). This relationship remained significant after adjustment for major cardiovascular risk factors, and each of four inflammatory markers (IL-6, CRP, ICAM-1 and fibrinogen). The largest evidence of mediation was for ICAM-1, but ICAM-1 levels explained only about 12% of the link between depression and cardiac events.

To summarize, available research suggests that it is likely that multiple overlapping and interacting mechanisms are involved in the link between depression and CAD. It is also probable that precise mechanisms vary from patient to patient. However, the number of studies that have assessed depression, potential mechanisms and cardiac events is limited, and, to date none have investigated the combined importance of several different behavioral and pathophysiological pathways. Much remains to be learned.

Conclusions

Interestingly, the same mechanisms that have been hypothesized to play a role in the relationship between depression and CAD have also been suggested to explain the impact of omega-3 fatty acid supplementation on cardiac events [38]. There is also evidence that stress and the chronic activation of the HPA axis, characteristic of depression, reduces the efficiency of the enzymes used to elongate and desaturate shorter and medium chain polyunsaturated fatty acids [39]. Considered in the light of our recent findings, described earlier, concerning reduced omega-3 levels associated with depression in CAD patients [25], and the promising results of several small trials of omega-3 supplementation as adjuvant treatment for depression in patients without CAD [40-42], additional mechanistic, as well as treatment studies of omega-3 fatty acids in depressed CAD patients, should clearly be part of the next generation of research concerning the complex interactions of brain, mind and heart.

References

[1]   C.J. Murray and A.D. Lopez. Global mortality, disability, and the contribution of risk factors: global burden of disease study. *Lancet* **349** (1997) 1436-1442.

[2]   American Psychiatric Association. Diagnostic and Statistical Manual of Mental Disorders, Fourth Edition. American Psychiatric Association Washington, D.C. (1994).

[3]   N. Frasure-Smith, F. Lespérance, M. Talajic. Depression and 18-month prognosis after myocardial infarction. *Circulation* **91** (1995) 999-1005.

[4]   F. Lespérance, N. Frasure-Smith, M. Juneau *et al.* Depression and 1-year prognosis in unstable angina. *Arch. Intern. Med.* **160** (2000) 1354-1360.

[5]   W. Jiang, J. Alexander, E. Christopher *et al.* Relationship of depression to increased risk of mortality and rehospitalization in patients with congestive heart failure. *Arch. Intern. Med.* **161** (2001) 1849-1856.

[6]   I. Connerney, P.A. Shapiro, J.S. McLaughlin *et al.* Relation between depression after coronary artery bypass surgery and 12-month outcome: a prospective study. *Lancet* **358** (2001) 1766-1771.

[7]   M. Hance, R.M. Carney, K.E. Freedland *et al.* Depression in patients with coronary heart disease: a 12-month follow-up. *Gen. Hosp. Psychiatry* **18** (1996) 61-65.

[8]   F. Lespérance and N. Frasure-Smith. Depression in patients with cardiac disease: a practical review. *J. Psychosom. Res.* **48** (2000) 379-391.

[9]   C. Sorensen, E. Friis-Hasche, T. Haghfelt *et al.* Postmyocardial infarction mortality in relation to depression: a systematic critical review. *Psychother. Psychosom.* **74** (2005) 69-80.

[10]   W.E. Narrow, D.S. Rae, L.N. Robins *et al.* Revised prevalence estimates of mental disorders in the United States: using a clinical significance criterion to reconcile 2 surveys' estimates. *Arch. Gen. Psychiatry* **59** (2002) 115-123.

[11]   R.M. Post. Transduction of psychosocial stress into the neurobiology of recurrent affective disorder. *Am. J. Psychiatry* **149** (1992) 999-1010.

[12]   F. Lespérance, N. Frasure-Smith, M. Talajic. Major depression before and after myocardial infarction: its nature and consequences. *Psychosom. Med.* **58** (1996) 99-110.

[13]   N. Frasure-Smith and F. Lespérance. Reflections on depression as a cardiac risk factor. *Psychosom. Med.* **67 Suppl. 1** (2005) S19-S25.

[14]   J. Barth, M. Schumacher, C. Herrmann-Lingen. Depression as a risk factor for mortality in patients with coronary heart disease: a meta-analysis. *Psychosom. Med.* **66** (2004) 802-813.

[15]   F. Lespérance, N. Frasure-Smith, M. Talajic *et al.* Five-year risk of cardiac mortality in relation to initial severity and one-year changes in depression symptoms after myocardial infarction. *Circulation* **105** (2002) 1049-1053.

[16]   R. Rugulies. Depression as a predictor for coronary heart disease. A review and meta-analysis. *Am. J. Prev. Med.* **23** (2002) 51-61.

[17]   S. Wassertheil-Smoller, S. Shumaker, J. Ockene *et al.* Depression and cardiovascular sequelae in postmenopausal women: the Women's Health Initiative (WHI). *Arch. Intern. Med.* **164** (2004) 289-298.

[18]   S. Yusuf, S. Hawken, S. Ounpuu *et al.* Effect of potentially modifiable risk factors associated with myocardial infarction in 52 countries (the INTERHEART study): case-control study. *Lancet* **364** (2004) 937-952.

[19]   N. Frasure-Smith and F. Lespérance. Depression and coronary heart disease: complex synergism of mind, body, and environment. *Current Directions in Psychological Science* **14** (2005) 39-43.

[20]   K.E. Joynt, D.J. Whellan, C.M. O'Connor. Depression and cardiovascular disease: mechanisms of interaction. *Biol. Psychiatry* **54** (2003) 248-261.

[21]   R.C. Ziegelstein, J.A. Fauerbach, S.S. Stevens *et al.* Patients with depression are less likely to follow recommendations to reduce cardiac risk during recovery from a myocardial infarction. *Arch. Intern. Med.* **160** (2000) 1818-1823.

[22]   R.M. Carney, K.E. Freedland, S.A. Eisen *et al.* Major depression and medication adherence in elderly patients with coronary artery disease. *Health Psychol.* **14** (1995) 88-90.

[23]   B.G. Druss, W.D. Bradford, R.A. Rosenheck *et al.* Quality of medical care and excess mortality in older patients with mental disorders. *Arch. Gen. Psychiatry* **58** (2001) 565-572.

[24]   R.M. Carney, J.A. Blumenthal, P.K. Stein *et al.* Depression, heart rate variability, and acute myocardial infarction. *Circulation* **104** (2001) 2024-2028.

[25]   F. Lespérance, N. Frasure-Smith, P. Theroux *et al.* The association between major depression and levels of soluble intercellular adhesion molecule 1, interleukin-6, and C-reactive protein in patients with recent acute coronary syndromes. *Am. J. Psychiatry* **161** (2004) 271-277.

[26]   E.P. Zorrilla, L. Luborsky, J.R. McKay *et al.* The relationship of depression and stressors to immunological assays: a meta-analytic review. *Brain Behav. Immun.* **15** (2001) 199-226.

[27]   S. Rajagopalan, R. Brook, M. Rubenfire *et al.* Abnormal brachial artery flow-mediated vasodilation in young adults with major depression. *Am. J. Cardiol.* **88** (2001) 196-198, A7.

[28]   A.J. Broadley, A. Korszun, C.J. Jones *et al.* Arterial endothelial function is impaired in treated depression. *Heart* **88** (2002) 521-523.

[29]   B.G. Pollock, F. Laghrissi-Thode, W.R. Wagner. Evaluation of platelet activation in depressed patients with ischemic heart disease after paroxetine or nortriptyline treatment. *J. Clin. Psychopharmacol.* **20** (2000) 137-140.

[30]   V.L. Serebruany, A.H. Glassman, A.I. Malinin *et al.* Enhanced platelet endothelial activation in depressed patients with acute coronary syndromes: evidence from recent clinical trials. *Blood Coagul. Fibrinolysis* **14** (2003) 563-567.

[31]   R. Edwards, M. Peet, J. Shay *et al.* Omega-3 polyunsaturated fatty acid levels in the diet and in red blood cell membranes of depressed patients. *J. Affect. Disord.* **48** (1998) 149-155.

[32]   M. Maes, A. Christophe, J. Delanghe *et al.* Lowered ω3 polyunsaturated fatty acids in serum phospholipids and cholesteryl esters of depressed patients. *Psychiatry Res.* **85** (1999) 275-291.

[33]   M. Maes, R. Smith, A. Christophe *et al.* Fatty acid composition in major depression: decreased ω3 fractions in cholesteryl esters and increased C20: 4ω6/C20:5ω3 ratio in cholesteryl esters and phospholipids. *J. Affect. Disord.* **38** (1996) 35-46.

[34]   H. Tiemeier, H.R. van Tuijl, A. Hofman *et al.* Plasma fatty acid composition and depression are associated in the elderly: the Rotterdam study. *Am. J. Clin. Nutr.* **78** (2003) 40-46.

[35]   N. Frasure-Smith, F. Lespérance, P. Julien. Major depression is associated with lower omega-3 fatty acid levels in patients with recent acute coronary syndromes. *Biol. Psychiatry* **55** (2004) 891-896.

[36]   R.M. Carney, J.A. Blumenthal, K.E. Freedland *et al.* Low heart rate variability and the effect of depression on post-myocardial infarction mortality. *Arch. Intern. Med.* **165** (2005) 1486-1491.

[37]   J.P. Empana, D.H. Sykes, G. Luc *et al.* Contributions of depressive mood and circulating inflammatory markers to coronary heart disease in healthy European men: the Prospective Epidemiological Study of Myocardial Infarction (PRIME). *Circulation* **111** (2005) 2299-2305.

[38]   B.J. Holub. Clinical nutrition: 4. Omega-3 fatty acids in cardiovascular care. *CMAJ* **166** (2002) 608-615.

[39]   J.R. Hibbeln and N. Salem Jr. Dietary polyunsaturated fatty acids and depression: when cholesterol does not satisfy. *Am. J. Clin. Nutr.* **62** (1995) 1-9.

[40]   B. Nemets, Z. Stahl, R.H. Belmaker. Addition of omega-3 fatty acid to maintenance medication treatment for recurrent unipolar depressive disorder. *Am. J. Psychiatry* **159** (2002) 477-479.

[41]   K.P. Su, S.Y. Huang, C.C. Chiu *et al.* Omega-3 fatty acids in major depressive disorder. A preliminary double-blind, placebo-controlled trial. *Eur. Neuropsychopharmacol.* **13** (2003) 267-271.

[42]   M. Peet and D.F. Horrobin. A dose-ranging study of the effects of ethyl-eicosapentaenoate in patients with ongoing depression despite apparently adequate treatment with standard drugs. *Arch. Gen. Psychiatry* **59** (2002) 913-919.

Effects of Omega-3 Polyunsaturated Fatty Acids on Depression

W. Emanuel Severus

Ludwig-Maximilians-University, Department of Psychiatry, Nußbaumstrasse 7,
80336 Munich, Germany

Abstract. Depression is characterised by depressed mood or/and the loss of interest or pleasure in nearly all activities for a substantial period of time, causing significant distress. Depression is a potentially life-threatening disease. It is a major risk factor for suicide as well as coronary artery disease (CAD) and sudden cardiac death (SCD). It also may be associated with impaired endothelial dysfunction and decreased heart rate variability (HRV). Both conditions seem to persist in patients with depression despite successful antidepressant treatment. During the last few years epidemiological studies as well as clinical trials have suggested a significant role of omega-3 fatty acids in the pathogenesis of depression. As omega-3 fatty acids have been demonstrated to also beneficially influence many of the conditions depression is a risk factor for (CAD, SCD) or may be associated with (decreased HRV, endothelial dysfunction), they may well represent a major advance in the treatment of depression. However more large randomized clinical trials are clearly needed to substantiate that claim.

Keywords. Affective disorders, cardiovascular diseases, omega-3 fatty acids

Effects of Omega-3 Polyunsaturated Fatty Acids on Depression

Depression (i.e. clinical depression, Major Depressive Disorder, depressive symptoms) is characterised by depressed mood or/and the loss of interest or pleasure in nearly activities. These symptoms have to persist for a significant duration of time, in the case of a major depressive episode for most of the day, nearly every day, for at least 2 consecutive weeks (DSM-IV). Furthermore they must cause clinically significant distress or impairment in social, occupational or other important areas of functioning. Other symptoms which often accompany depressed mood and loss of interest or pleasure include, among others, difficulties to concentrate, to make decisions, sleeping difficulties (early awakening or hypersomnia), changes in appetite or weight, low self-esteem, sometimes mounting to feelings of worthlessness or guilt and thoughts of death, suicidal ideation and suicide.

Dependent on the severity of the illness psychotropic drugs and/or psychotherapy (e.g. cognitive behavioural therapy) are the treatment of choice. There are different groups of antidepressants, each with several members, which are approved for the treatment of depression. Using these drugs the majority of individuals suffering from depression can be successfully treated, allowing them to lead normal lives with little impairment.

However, depression is a systemic disease, associated with substantially increased "medical" morbidity and mortality.

Depression is the main risk factor for committing suicide, with approximately 10% of subjects with recurrent depressive disorder dying of it [1]. While antidepressants, and in particular lithium, are able to partially decrease that risk, even patients with treated depression commit suicide [2].

Depression is a major independent risk factor for developing coronary artery disease and myocardial infarction [3-5]. Once the coronary artery disease is present individuals with depression are at an increased risk of suffering a fatal cardiac event [6-8]. Increased abdominal fat deposition [9,10], decreased heart rate variability [11] and impaired arterial endothelial function, which even persists after the successful antidepressant treatment of depression, including SSRIs, seem to account for this phenomenon, at least partially [12,13].

Two prospective randomized, double-blind, placebo/usual care-controlled multicenter trials have studied the impact of antidepressants and psychotherapy/antidepressants in patients with myocardial infarction/unstable angina and depression.

- In SADHART (Sertraline Antidepressant Heart Attack Randomized Trial), 369 patients with Major Depressive Disorder (64% male; mean age, 57.1 years; mean 17-item Hamilton Depression [HAM-D] score, 19.6; MI, 74%; unstable angina, 26%) were randomly assigned to receive sertraline in flexible dosages of 50 to 200 mg/d (n = 186) or placebo (n = 183) for 24 weeks. While sertraline was safe and effective in the treatment of the affective symptoms of depression (especially in those with severe or recurrent Major Depressive Disorder) it had no significant effect on cardiovascular risk factors, such as left ventricular ejection fraction, treatment-emergent increase in ventricular premature complex (VPC) runs, QTc-interval greater than 450 milliseconds at end-point or other cardiac measures, including heart rate variability. The incidence of severe cardiovascular adverse events was 14.5% with sertraline and 22.4% with placebo [14].

- In the ENRICHD (Enhancing Recovery in Coronary Heart Disease Patients) trial 2481 MI patients (1084 women, 1397 men) were randomly allocated to usual medical care or Cognitive behavioural therapy-based psychosocial intervention. Cognitive behaviour therapy was initiated for a median of 11 individual sessions throughout 6 months, plus group therapy when feasible, with SSRIs for patients scoring higher than 24 on the Hamilton Rating Scale of Depression (HRSD) or having a less than 50% reduction in Beck Depression Inventory scores after 5 weeks. After an average follow-up of 29 months, there was no significant difference in event-free survival between usual care (75.9%) and psychosocial intervention (75.8%). There were also no differences in survival between the psychosocial intervention and usual care arms in any of the 3 psychosocial risk groups (depression, low perceived social support (LPSS), and depression and LPSS patients) [15]. However, in an uncontrolled post-hoc observation, the risk of death or recurrent MI was significantly lower in patients taking selective serotonin reuptake inhibitors (adjusted HR, 0.57; CI 0.38 - 084), as were the risk of all-cause mortality (adjusted HR, 0.59; 95% CI, 0.37 - 0.96) and recurrent MI (adjusted HR, 0.53; 95% CI: 0.32 - 0.90), compared with patients who did not take SSRIs [16].

While both intervention trials had no statistically significant effect on cardiovascular events in the overall sample, SSRIs may decrease the risk of cardiovascular events in those patients with more severe illness. However, some risk factors for coronary artery disease, such as impaired endothelial function [12,13] or decreased heart rate variability, which seems to be present in a substantial number [17], but not all patients with depression and coronary artery disease [18], may persist despite successful antidepressant treatment. Consequently the increased rates of cardiovascular disease in patients with depression may, at least partially, be a trait marker of depression. Alternatively, they may be the result of a still unrecognized underlying physiological factor that predisposes an individual to both depression and cardiovascular disease [19].

If this were true, this underlying physiological factor should remain unchanged even after successful treatment of depression with antidepressants. Furthermore it should be associated with risk factors for cardiovascular morbidity/mortality, such as impaired endothelial function, present in treated depression.

One such candidate may be a functional deficit of omega-3 fatty acids [20].

Omega-3 fatty acids are essential polyunsaturated fatty acids, with alpha-linolenic acid (ALA), eicosapentaenoic acid (EPA) and docosahexaenoic acid (DHA) being the most important representatives. While the main dietary source of ALA is flaxseed oil, EPA and DHA can be most abundantly found in wild-bred fatty fish, such as herring, mackerel, salmon and tuna.

Several lines of evidence point to a possible involvement of omega-3 fatty acids in depression.

- Patient-based as well as population-based case-control studies have repeatedly shown that depression is associated with lower omega-3 fatty acids and an increased ratio of omega-6 PUFAs/omega-3 PUFAs, AA/EPA and AA/DHA in red blood cell phospholipids and plasma phospholipids, respectively (see Table 1 for details). This observation has been made in patients with [21] and without comorbid coronary artery disease [22-25]. Furthermore, the successful treatment of depression with antidepressants does not significantly change this association [24]. Decreased dietary intake [23] as well as increased oxidative stress seems to account for this phenomenon [24].
- Having in mind that omega-3 fatty acids are effective in and approved for the treatment of hypertriglyceridaemia ("OMACOR®"), it is of particular interest that patients with depression and recent coronary syndromes have increased triglyceride levels compared with patients with recent coronary syndromes but without comorbid depression [21].
- Epidemiological data show that nations with high fish consumption have significantly lower rates of major depression (r = -0.84, p<0.005) [26].
- Double-blind, placebo-controlled studies have shown that omega-3 fatty acids improve risk factors for coronary artery (decreased heart rate variability [27,28], impaired arterial endothelial function [29]) which may persist in successfully treated depression.
- In animal models of depression omega-3 fatty acids have similar properties as approved conventional antidepressants [30]. Furthermore supplementation with omega-3 fatty acids at clinically relevant doses leads to significant changes in major neurotransmitters in the brain, intimately involved in mood regulation [31].

Table 1. Selected studies of omega-3 fatty acids and affective disorders (adapted and extended from Severus *et al* (2001) [20]

Study	Subjects	Study design/methods	Results
Adams *et al*, 1996 [22]	20 in- and outpatients with DSM-IV unipolar depression (all but 3 drug-free), HAM-D scores 14.5-36	Clinical study. Dietary intake of lipids over the previous 3 mo assessed with the Food Frequency Questionnaire; RBC phospholipids and plasma PUFA levels measured; severity of depression determined with the 21-item HAM-D and a linear rating scale.	RBC phospholipid AA:EPA ratio was positively correlated with the severity of depression, measured with the HAM-D ($r = 0.472$, $p<0.05$) and the linear rating scale ($r = 0.729$, $p<0.001$); RBC phospholipid EPA level was negatively correlated with the severity of depression, measured with the linear rating scale ($r = -0.546$, $p<0.005$). No significant correlations were found between estimated EPA intake from fish and either REC EPA level or RBC AA:EPA ratio.
Edwards *et al*, 1998 [23]	10 patients with major depressive episode, all taking antidepressant medication, and 14 healthy age- and gender-matched controls	Controlled clinical study. All subjects assessed with the BDI, current diet assessed with the 7-d weighed intake method; RBC membrane omega-3 fatty acids, omega-6 fatty acids, and saturated and monounsaturated fatty acids measured.	Patients showed a significant decrease in RBC membrane n-3 PUFA levels (EPA, p=0.02; DHA, p=0.02; total n-3, p=0.02) compared to controls but no significant abnormalities in n-6 PUFAs. Smoking and recent stressful life events had no significant effect on RBC membrane levels of individual or total n-3 fatty acids. Patients and controls did not differ significantly in current dietary intake of n-3 fatty acids or total energy intake. Among the depressed patients, dietary ALA (r = -0.83, p=0.003) and RBC membrane ALA (r = -0.81, p=0.008) were the only strong predictors of BDI scores.
Peet *et al*, 1998 [24]	15 patients with a DSM-IV major depressive episode (unipolar illness), free of psychotropic medication for at least 7 d (mean, 16.7 ± 20 days), and 15 healthy age- and gender-matched controls	Controlled clinical study. Comparison of RBC membrane fatty acid levels in patients and controls. A second blood sample was drawn from 10 of the patients after 6 weeks of antidepressant treatment with lofepramine or amisulpride.	Patients showed a significant depletion in RBC membrane fatty acid levels of DHA (p=0.009), DPA (p=0.04), total n-3 (p=0.02), linoleic acid (p=0.005), DGLA (p=0.02), and total n-6 (p=0.02) compared to controls. Patients also had non-significantly elevated AA:EPA and AA:DHA ratios (p=0.02 and 0.06, respectively) and significantly elevated levels of oleic acid (p=0.001), palmitic acid (p=0.03), and stearic acid (p=0.02) compared with controls. Patients, both before and after treatment, had lower DHA (F=4.0, p=0.03) and total RBC n-3 (F=3.61, p=0.04) levels than did controls; the difference disappeared after incubation of RBC with hydrogen peroxide in controls.

Study	Subjects	Study design/methods	Results
Frasure-Smith *et al*, 2004 [21]	54 cases with a DSM-IV major depressive episode (unipolar illness), one third taking antidepressants (all SSRIs) and 54 sex- and age-matched controls: cases and controls were hospitalized for an acute coronary syndrome approximately 2 months before the assessment	Case control study. Comparison of plasma phospholipids PUFAs. Assessment of numerous co-variates.	Cases showed a significant decrease of DHA (p=0.013; effect size: 0.53), total EPA + DHA (p=0.024) and total n-3 (p=0.44; effect size: 0.37), compared to controls. Cases showed a significant increase of two omega-6 fatty acids, i.e. gamma-linoleic acid (p=0.011) and adrenic acid (p=0.001), compared to controls. Cases had significantly elevated ratios of n-6/n-3 (p=0.044), AA/EPA (p=0.044) and AA/DHA (p=0.002) compared to controls. Regarding co-variates cases differed from controls in having significantly increased fasting triglycerides (p=0.005).
Tiemeier et al, 2003 [25]	264 subjects aged ≥60 years with depressive symptoms, including 106 subjects with depressive disorders; 461 randomly selected reference subjects	Population-based case-control study. Comparison of plasma phospholipids and their ratios between the different groups.	Subjects with depressive disorders had a higher ratio of n-6/n-3 PUFAs (p=0.05) and AA/DHA (p=0.04), but not AA/EPA (p=0.06). These differences became more pronounced when only depressed subjects with low CRP concentrations were considered (n-6/n-3 PUFAs: p=0.0006; AA/EPA: p=0.007; AA/DHA: p=0.02).

AA, arachidonic acid; *ALA*, alpha-linolenic acid; *BDI*, Beck Depression Inventory; *DGLA*, dihomogammalinolenic acid; *DHA*, docosahexaenoic acid; *DPA*, docosapentaenoic acid; *DSM-IV*, Diagnostic and Statistical Manual of Mental Disorders, 4th edition; *EPA*, eicosapentaenoic acid; *HAM-D*, Hamilton Rating Scale for Depression; *PUFA*, polyunsaturated fatty acid; *RBC*, red blood cell; *YMRS*, Young Mania Rating Scale.

A functional deficit of omega-3 fatty acids may also contribute to suicidal thoughts, suicide attempts and completed suicides. This is of importance as depression is the main risk factor for all three areas:

- In a case-control study, red blood cell EPA and DHA levels were significantly lower in individuals having attempted suicide than in patients injured by accidents (EPA: $p<0.0001$; DHA: $p<0.0003$). When the highest and lowest quartiles of EPA and DHA in RBC were compared, the odds ratios of suicide attempt was 0.12 in the highest quartile (95% CI: 0.04 - 0.36, p for trend=0.0001) after adjustment for possible confounding factors [32].

- Suicides and suspected suicides, as well as sudden cardiac death, but not accident victims, are accompanied by a high ratio of 20:4 n-6/22:6 n-3 in autopsy samples from heart muscle [33].

- In a population-based case-control study both the risk of being depressed and the risk of having suicidal ideation were significantly lower among frequent lake-fish consumers compared with more infrequent consumers after adjusting for potential confounders [34]. However, another study [35] could not confirm these results.

The above observations have let researchers to initiate double-blind, controlled trials of omega-3 fatty acids (EPA, DHA, EPA/DHA) in depression/mood disorders (see Tables 2, 3 and 4 for details). Most of the trials were add-on trials with omega-3 fatty acids or placebo added to ongoing antidepressant treatment [36-38]). All studies, except one trial [39], were acute treatment trials. Study duration was between 4 weeks [38] and 4 months [39].

Table 2. EPA in depression

Study	Mental Disorder	Dose, number of subjects	Study duration	Monotherapy? Add-on?	Results
Peet & Horrobin, 2002 [36]	Unipolar Depression	1 g EPA: N = 17	12 weeks	Add-on	1 g EPA > Placebo
		2 g EPA: N = 18			2 g EPA = Placebo
		4 g EPA: N = 17			4 g EPA = Placebo
		Placebo: N = 18			
Frangou & Lewis, 2002 [37]	Bipolar Depression	1 g EPA: N = 24	12 weeks	Add-on	EPA > Placebo
		2 g EPA: N = 25			1 g EPA = 2 g EPA
		Placebo: N = 26			
Nemets *et al*, 2002 [38]	Major Depressive Disorder, recurrent	2 g EPA: N = 10	4 weeks	Add-on	2 g EPA > Placebo
		Placebo: N = 10			
Zanarini & Frankenburg, 2003 [40]	Depression (Borderline Personality Disorder)	1 g EPA: N = 20	8 weeks	Monotherapy	1 g EPA > Placebo
		Placebo: N = 10			
Post/Keck *et al*, 2003 [41]	Bipolar Depression	6 g EPA, Placebo: N = 59	4 months	Add-on	6 g EPA = Placebo

Most studies used pure Ethyl-EPA at doses between 1 to 6 g/day [36-38,40,41]. Pure DHA was used between 1 and 4 g/day [42,43].

Table 3. DHA in depression

Study	Mental Disorder	Dose, number of subjects	Study duration	Monotherapy? Add-on?	Results
Mischoulon *et al*, 2004 [43]	Major Depressive Disorder	1 g DHA: N = 14	12 weeks	Monotherapy	Response rate (ITT):
		2 g DHA: N = 10			1 g = 45%
		4 g DHA: N = 10			2 g = 33%
					4 g = 0%
Marangell *et al*, 2003 [42]	Major Depressive Disorder	2 g DHA: N = 18	6 weeks	Monotherapy	DHA=
		Placebo: N = 17			Placebo

Two studies used a combination of EPA/DHA (EPA>DHA) at 6.6 [44] and 9.6 g/day [39], respectively.

Table 4. EPA/DHA in depression

Study	Mental Disorder	Dose, number of subjects	Study duration	Monotherapy? Add-on?	Results
Stoll *et al*, 1999 [39]	Bipolar Disorder (Manic Depressive Illness)	6.2 g EPA + 3.4 g DHA: N = 14	4 months	Add-on	EPA/DHA > placebo regarding survival in study, antidepressant properties
		Placebo: N = 16		N = 8 (Monotherapy)	
Su *et al*, 2003 [44]	Major Depressive Disorder	4.4 g EPA + 2.2 g DHA: N = 12	8 weeks	Add-on	EPA/DHA > placebo
		Placebo: N = 10			

Subjects taking part in these trials were suffering from depressive symptoms in the context of unipolar depression [36], Major Depressive Disorder [38,42-44], bipolar disorder [37,39,41] or borderline personality disorder [40]. The studies were without exception small trials, with 20 [38] to 75 subjects [37] taking part in it.

With the exception of one trial [42], no baseline assessment of plasma or red blood cell phospholipids PUFAs was performed (or published). The results can be summarized as follows:

- There are 2 studies showing significant antidepressant properties of 1 g of Ethyl-EPA compared to placebo (monotherapy, add-on treatment) [36,40]. In another trial in bipolar depression, the combined data of 1 and 2 g of Ethyl-EPA showed significantly superior antidepressant properties of EPA compared to placebo, with 1 g EPA being as effective as 2 g of EPA [37]. However there is also a negative study showing no significant difference of 2 g of Ethyl-EPA compared to placebo in unipolar depression [36]. Similarly 4 and 6 g of EPA did not perform better than placebo (unipolar depression, bipolar depression) [36,41].

- 2 g of DHA were no more effective than placebo in unipolar depression [42]. The subjects however showed no signs of an omega-3 fatty acids deficiency at baseline (red blood cells). In another randomized controlled trial, 1 g of DHA was significantly superior to 4 g of DHA, however there was no placebo group in this trial [43].

- 6.6 and 9.6 g of a combination of EPA and DHA showed significantly superior antidepressant properties compared to placebo in the acute treatment of unipolar depression [44] and the prophylactic treatment of bipolar disorder [39]. No trials with lower doses of this combination have been performed/published.

There are no controlled trials of ALA in depression. An open study (N = 3, on-off-design) however suggests that flaxseed oil is able to improve depressive symptoms in Major Depressive Disorder (2.5 tablespoons) and trigger manic episodes in unipolar and bipolar depression at higher doses (5 tablespoons), which hints at significant antidepressant properties of flaxseed oil [45].

The clinician inclined to use omega-3 fatty acids in the treatment of depression encounters the following obstacles:

- No drug containing omega-3 fatty is approved for the treatment of depression worldwide.

- No trial of "OMACOR®" - the only drug containing omega-3 fatty acids approved in Europe (for secondary prevention of myocardial infarction and for the treatment of hypertriglyeridaemia) - has been performed in individuals with depression. In "OMACOR®" the ratio of EPA to DHA is similar to, but not identical to the study drugs, used in both EPA/DHA combination trials, yielding positive results.

- Ethyl-EPA, the drug with the best evidence for antidepressant properties, is only licensed in Japan.

Therefore, at present, unless randomized controlled trials of "OMACOR®" in patients with depression (and past myocardial infarction or hypertriglyceridaemia) have been conducted, "OMACOR®" should only be used in patients with depression and comorbid coronary artery disease or hypertriglyceridaemia, at the appropriate dose according to the primary condition, i.e.:

- Secondary prevention after myocardial infarction: 1 capsule/day
- Hypertriglyeridaemia: 2(-4) capsules/day.

In these cases however, due to the huge potential benefits of these fatty acids in depression, the use of "OMACOR®" is highly recommended.

References

[1]   J. Licinio and M.L. Wong. Depression, antidepressants and suicidality: a critical appraisal. *Nat. Rev. Drug Discov.* **4** (2005) 165-171.

[2]   D. Fergusson, S. Doucette, K.C. Glass *et al.* Association between suicide attempts and selective serotonin reuptake inhibitors: systematic review of randomised controlled trials. *BMJ* **330** (2005) 396.

[3]   J.C. Barefoot and M. Schroll. Symptoms of depression, acute myocardial infarction, and total mortality in a community sample. *Circulation* **93** (1996) 1976-1980.

[4]   L.A. Pratt, D.E. Ford, R.M. Crum *et al.* Depression, psychotropic medication, and risk of myocardial infarction. Prospective data from the Baltimore ECA follow-up. *Circulation* **94** (1996) 3123-3129.

[5]   D.E. Ford, L.A. Mead, P.P. Chang *et al.* Depression is a risk factor for coronary artery disease in men: the precursors study. *Arch. Intern. Med.* **158** (1998) 1422-1426.

[6]   R.M. Carney, M.W. Rich, K.E. Freedland *et al.* Major depressive disorder predicts cardiac events in patients with coronary artery disease. *Psychosom. Med.* **50** (1988) 627-633.

[7]   J.C. Barefoot, M.J. Helms, D.B. Mark *et al.* Depression and long-term mortality risk in patients with coronary artery disease. *Am. J. Cardiol.* **78** (1996) 613-617.

[8]   N. Frasure-Smith, T. Lespérance, M. Talajic. Depression and 18-month prognosis after myocardial infarction. *Circulation* **91** (1995) 999-1005.

[9]   J.H. Thakore, P.J. Richards, R.H. Reznek *et al.* Increased intra-abdominal fat deposition in patients with major depressive illness as measured by computed tomography. *Biol Psychiatry* **41** (1997) 1140-1142.

[10]   B. Weber-Hamann, F. Hentschel, A. Kniest *et al.* Hypercortisolemic depression is associated with increased intra-abdominal fat. *Psychosom. Med.* **64** (2002) 274-277.

[11]   R.M. Carney, J.A. Blumenthal, K.E. Freedland *et al.* Low heart rate variability and the effect of depression on post-myocardial infarction mortality. *Arch. Intern. Med.* **165** (2005) 1486-1491.

[12]   S. Rajagopalan, R. Brook, M. Rubenfire *et al.* Abnormal brachial artery flow-mediated vasodilation in young adults with major depression. *Am. J. Cardiol.* **88** (2001) 196-198.

[13]   A.J. Broadley, A. Korszun, C.J. Jones *et al.* Arterial endothelial function is impaired in treated depression. *Heart* **88** (2002) 521-523.

[14]   A.H. Glassman, C.M. O'Connor, R.M. Califf *et al.* Sertraline treatment of major depression in patients with acute MI or unstable angina. *JAMA* **288** (2002) 701-709.

[15]   L.F. Berkman, J. Blumenthal, M. Burg *et al.* Effects of treating depression and low perceived social support on clinical events after myocardial infarction: the Enhancing Recovery in Coronary Heart Disease Patients (ENRICHD) Randomized Trial. *JAMA* **289** (2003) 3106-3116.

[16]   C.B. Taylor, M.E. Youngblood, D. Catellier *et al.* Effects of the antidepressant medication in morbidity and mortality in depressed patients after myocardial infarction. *Arch. Gen. Psychiatry* **62** (2005) 792-798.

[17]   P.K. Stein, R.M. Carney, K.E. Freedland *et al.* Severe depression is associated with markedly reduced heart rate variability in patients with stable coronary artery disease. *J. Psychosom. Res.* **48** (2000) 493-500.

[18]   A. Gehi, D. Mangano, S. Pipkin *et al.* Depression and heart rate variability in patients with stable coronary heart disease: findings from the Heart and Soul Study. *Arch. Gen. Psychiatry* **62** (2005) 661-666.

[19]   F. Lespérance and N. Frasure-Smith. The seduction of death. *Psychosom. Med.* **61** (1999) 18-20.

[20]   W.E. Severus, A.B. Littman, A.L. Stoll. Omega-3 fatty acids, homocysteine, and the increased risk of cardiovascular mortality in major depressive disorder. *Harv. Rev. Psychiatry* **9** (2001) 280-293.

[21]   N. Frasure-Smith, F. Lespérance, P. Julien. Major depression is associated with lower omega-3 fatty acid levels in patients with recent acute coronary syndromes. *Biol. Psychiatry* **55** (2004) 891-896.

[22]   P.B. Adams, S. Lawson, A. Sanigorski *et al.* Arachidonic acid to eicosapentaenoic acid ratio in blood correlates positively with clinical symptoms of depression. *Lipids* **31** (1996) S157-S161.

[23]   R. Edwards, M. Peet, J. Shay *et al.* Omega-3 polyunsaturated fatty acid levels in the diet and in red blood cell membranes of depressed patients. *J. Affect. Disord.* **48** (1998) 149-155.

[24]   M. Peet, B. Murphy, J. Shay *et al.* Depletion of omega-3 fatty acid levels in red blood cell membranes of depressive patients. *Biol Psychiatry* **43** (1998) 315-319.

[25]   H. Tiemeier, H.R. van Tuijl, A. Hofman *et al.* Plasma fatty acid composition and depression are associated in the elderly: the Rotterdam Study. *Am. J. Clin. Nutr.* **78** (2003) 40-46.

[26]   J.R. Hibbeln. Fish consumption and major depression. *Lancet* **351** (1998) 1213.

[27]   B. Villa, L. Calabresi, G. Chiesa *et al.* Omega-3 fatty acid ethyl esters increase heart rate variability in patients with coronary disease. *Pharmacol. Res.* **45** (2002) 475.

[28]   J.H. Christensen, P. Gustenhoff, E. Korup *et al.* Effect of fish oil on heart rate variability in survivors of myocardial infarction: a double-blind randomised controlled trial. *BMJ* **312** (1996) 677-678.

[29]   J. Goodfellow, M.F. Bellamy, M.W. Ramsey *et al.* Dietary supplementation with marine omega-3 fatty acids improve systemic large artery endothelial function in subjects with hypercholesterolemia. *J. Am. Coll. Cardiol.* **35** (2000) 265-270.

[30]   W.A. Carlezon Jr, S.D. Mague, A.M. Parow *et al.* Antidepressant-like effects of uridine and omega-3 fatty acids are potentiated by combined treatment in rats. *Biol. Psychiatry* **57** (2005) 343-350.

[31]   S. Chalon, S. Vancassel, L. Zimmer *et al.* Polyunsaturated fatty acids and cerebral function: focus on monoaminergic neurotransmission. *Lipids* **36** (2001) 937-944.

[32]   M. Huan, K. Hamazaki, Y. Sun *et al.* Suicide attempt and n-3 fatty acid levels in red blood cells: a case control study in China. *Biol. Psychiatry* **56** (2004) 490-496.

[33]   S. Gudbjarnason. Dynamics of n-3 and n-6 fatty acids in phospholipids of heart muscle. *J. Intern. Med. Suppl.* **731** (1989) 117-128.

[34]   A. Tanskanen, J.R. Hibbeln, J. Hintikka *et al.* Fish consumption, depression, and suicidality in a general population. *Arch. Gen. Psychiatry* **58** (2001) 512-513.

[35]   R. Hakkarainen, T. Partonen, J. Haukka *et al.* Is low dietary intake of omega-3 fatty acids associated with depression? *Am. J. Psychiatry* **161** (2004) 567-569.

[36]   M. Peet and D.F. Horrobin. A dose-ranging study of the effects of ethyl-eicosapentaenoate in patients with ongoing depression despite apparently adequate treatment with standard drugs. *Arch. Gen. Psychiatry* **59** (2002) 913-919.

[37]　S. Frangou, M. Lewis, P. McCrone. Efficacy of ethyl-eicosapentaenoic acid in bipolar depression: randomised double-blind placebo-controlled study. *Br. J. Psychiatry* **188** (2006) 46-50.

[38]　B. Nemets, Z. Stahl, R.H. Belmaker. Addition of omega-3 fatty acid to maintenance medication treatment for recurrent unipolar depressive disorder. *Am. J. Psychiatry* **159** (2002) 477-479.

[39]　A.L. Stoll, W.E. Severus, M.P. Freeman *et al.* Omega 3 fatty acids in bipolar disorder: a preliminary double-blind, placebo-controlled trial. *Arch. Gen. Psychiatry* **56** (1999) 407-412.

[40]　M.C. Zanarini and F.R. Frankenburg. Omega-3 fatty acid treatment of women with borderline personality disorder: a double-blind, placebo-controlled pilot study. *Am. J. Psychiatry* **160** (2003) 167-169.

[41]　R.M. Post, G.S. Leverich, L.L. Altshuler *et al.* An overview of recent findings of the Stanley Foundation Bipolar Network (Part I). *Bipolar Disord.* **5** (2003) 310-319.

[42]　L.B. Marangell, J.M. Martinez, H.A. Zboyan *et al.* A double-blind, placebo-controlled study of the omega-3 fatty acid docosahexaenoic acid in the treatment of major depression. *Am. J. Psychiatry* **160** (2003) 996-998.

[43]　D. Mischoulon, J. Murakami, Y. Mahal *et al.* Double-blind dose-finding study of docosahexaenoic acid (DHA) in major depressive disorder. *NCDEU* (2004) Poster 193.

[44]　K.P. Su, S.Y. Huang, C.C. Chiu *et al.* Omega-3 fatty acids in major depressive disorder. A preliminary double-blind, placebo-controlled trial. *Eur. Neuropsychopharmacol.* **13** (2003) 267-271.

[45]　D.O. Rudin. The major psychoses and neuroses as omega-3 essential fatty acid deficiency syndrome: substrate pellagra. *Biol. Psychiatry* **16** (1981) 837-850.

A Multi-Country Health-Economic Evaluation of Highly Concentrated n-3 Polyunsaturated Fatty Acids (PUFAs) in the Secondary Prevention after Myocardial Infarction (MI)

Mark Lamotte[a], Lieven Annemans[a,b], Pawel Kawalec[c,d] and York Zoellner[e]

[a] *HEDM-IMS, Rue De Crayer 6, 1000 Brussels, Belgium*
[b] *Ghent University, Sint-Pietersnieuwstraat 25, 9000 Ghent, Belgium*
[c] *HTA Center, Nuszkiewicza Street 13/19, Krakow, Poland*
[d] *Institute of Public Health, Collegium Medium, Jagiellonian University, Grzegorzecka Street 20, Krakow, Poland*
[e] *Solvay Pharmaceuticals GmbH, Global Health Economics, P.O. Box 220, D-30002 Hannover, Germany*

Abstract. Patients who survive an acute myocardial infarction (MI) are at increased risk of subsequent major cardiovascular events and cardiac (often sudden) death. The use of highly concentrated and purified omega-3 polyunsaturated fatty acids (n-3 PUFAs), in addition to standard secondary prevention after MI, results in a significant reduction in the risk of sudden death. This study assessed the cost-effectiveness of adding n-3 PUFAs to the current secondary prevention treatment after acute MI in 5 countries: Australia, Belgium, Canada, Germany, Poland.

Based on the clinical outcomes of GISSI-Prevenzione (MI, stroke, revascularisation rate and mortality), a decision-model was built in DataPRO™. The implications of adding n-3 PUFAs to standard treatment in patients with a recent history of MI were analysed from the health care payer's perspective. The time horizon was 3.5 years (identical to GISSI-Prevenzione). Event costs were based on literature data. Life expectancy data for survivors of cardiac disease were taken from the Saskatchewan database and then country-adjusted. Results are expressed as extra cost (€) per life-year gained (LYG). Annual discounting of 5% was applied to health effects and costs.

Treatment with highly concentrated n-3 PUFAs yielded between 0.260 (Poland) and 0.284 (Australia) LYG, at an additional cost of € 807 (Canada) to € 1,451 (Belgium). The incremental cost-effectiveness ratio (ICER) varied between € 2,867 (Canada) and € 5,154 (Belgium) per LYG. Sensitivity analyses on effectiveness, cost of complications and discounting proved the robustness of the results. A 2nd order Monte Carlo simulation based on the 95% CIs obtained from GISSI showed that highly concentrated n-3 PUFAs are cost-effective in more than 99% of patients (assuming societal willingness to pay threshold of € 20,000/LYG). Including health care costs incurred during the remaining life-years considerably increased total costs, but had no impact on the ICER-based treatment recommendation.

Adding highly concentrated n-3 PUFAs to standard treatment in the secondary prevention after MI appears to be cost-effective in the 5 countries studied.

Keywords. Cost-effectiveness, myocardial infarction, sudden death, n-3 PUFA

Introduction

Enormous progress has been made in the management of acute myocardial infarction (MI) in the past 35 years [1]. Patients who have survived an acute MI are, nevertheless, a high-risk group with a life expectancy half that of their peers who have not experienced a similar event [2], and with a greatly increased risk of subsequent major cardiovascular events and death [3],[4]. Sudden cardiac death is a major contributor to this situation [5]. Sudden death has proven resistant to therapeutic innovation to a greater degree than atherothrombotic coronary disease. Incidence rates of sudden death post-MI have declined during the era of thrombolytic therapy but remain important. Nearly half the cardiovascular deaths in the USA are attributed to this cause [6],[7]. The current expert perspective on sudden death related to coronary disease is that it is "the single most important cause of death in the adult population of the industrialized world" [8].

The need for an effective, easy-to-use, broadly applicable and affordable medical therapy to prevent cardiovascular death and, in particular, sudden death is thus clear. A candidate therapy has emerged in the form of highly concentrated and purified omega-3 polyunsaturated fatty acids (omega-3 [or n-3] PUFAs). In the Gruppo Italiano per lo Studio della Sopravvivenza dell'Infarto Miocardico-Prevenzione trial (GISSI-P) study, use of n-3 PUFAs at a dose of 900 mg/day in addition to standard prevention was associated with a 45% reduction in risk of sudden death [9].

The aim of this study was to assess the cost-effectiveness of adding n-3 PUFA treatment to the current secondary prevention treatment after acute MI in five different countries, namely Australia, Belgium, Canada, Germany and Poland. A secondary objective was to estimate for the different countries the budget impact of administering highly concentrated n-3 PUFAs to all patients with a history of a recent MI.

1.   Methods

1.1.   Model Structure

A decision-tree was developed using the decision-analytic software DataPRO™ from TreeAge. The decision-tree simulates the current secondary prevention strategy as compared to a strategy including n-3 PUFAs. The model is based on the 3.5 years' outcome in the GISSI-P study. A graphical presentation of the model is shown in Figure 1.

In the model, the patient can be treated with or without n-3 PUFAs; in both cases, the patient has a risk of MI, stroke or a revascularisation, or the patient can die from a cardiovascular or non-cardiovascular cause as reported in GISSI-P (see further and Table 1) [9]. Both significant and non-significant differences were taken into account. Taking into account non-significant differences does not systematically favour treatment with n-3 PUFAs, as for example slightly more percutaneous interventions were performed and more strokes were reported in the n-3 PUFA arm resulting in higher costs.

The follow-up in the GISSI-P trial was 42 months (3.5 years). It is assumed that an event took place after an average of 1.75 years of follow-up. This is important for the discounting of future costs and for the calculation of the number of life-years gained with each strategy.

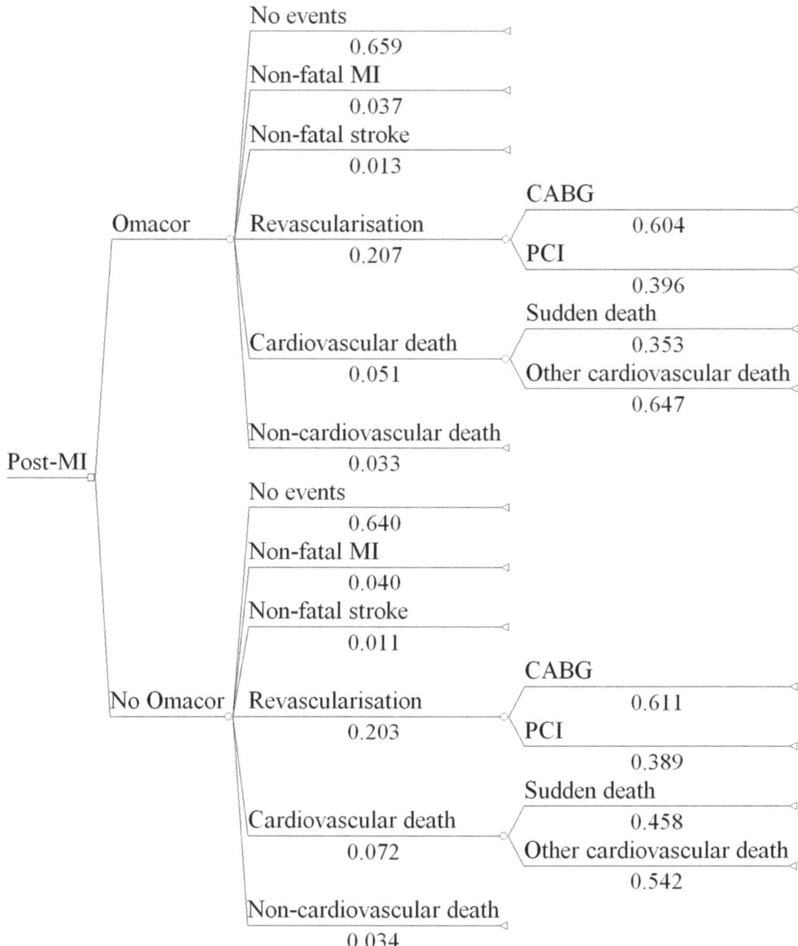

Figure 1. Structure of the model.

A country specific discount rate was applied to future costs and effects. Based on the latest information available on the website of the International Society of Pharmacoeconomics and Outcomes Research (September 2005; http://www.ispor.org/PEguidelines/) the discount rate to be applied is 5% for the 5 countries. The perspective of the third-party payer was taken. This perspective was chosen to show the possible benefits for the health care payer of reimbursing n-3 PUFAs. Therefore, only reimbursed medical costs are taken into account. Indirect costs are not considered.

The time horizon of the model is 3.5 years, but effects on life expectancy are calculated lifelong. According to the recommendations from several health economists (see for instance Johannesson *et al* [10]) costs of future life were also taken into account in this lifetime horizon.

1.2. Clinical Data

The largest long-term trial on highly concentrated n-3 polyunsaturated fatty acids was conducted by the GISSI-Prevenzione Investigators [9],[11],[12]. In this study, patients surviving a recent (≤3 months) MI were treated with either 900mg of highly concentrated n-3 PUFAs (n = 2836), 300 mg of vitamin E (n = 2830), a combination of both (n = 2830) or none of either (n = 2828). There were no baseline differences in patient characteristics. Patients were recommended to continue other preventive treatments such as aspirin, β-blockers and ACE-inhibitors. After 42 months of follow-up, a statistically significant difference in mortality between the placebo group and the group of patients treated with n-3 PUFAs (see Table 1) could be detected. This difference was entirely due to decreased cardiac death and, in particular, sudden death.

Table 1. Outcomes reported in the GISSI-Prevenzione study [9],[11],[12]

Event*	n-3 PUFAs (n = 2835)	Control (n = 2828)	RR (95% CI)
Total mortality	8.4	10.6	0.80 (0.67-0.94)
Non-CVD	2.1	1.6	1.35 (0.91-1.98)
Unknown	1.2	1.8	0.68 (0.44-1.04)
CVD‡	*5.1*	*7.2*	*0.70 (0.56-0.86)*
Cardiac death	*4.0*	*6.1*	*0.65 (0.51-0.82)*
Sudden death	*1.8*	*3.3*	*0.56 (0.40-0.79)*
Non-fatal events	4.9	4.9	0.98 (0.78-1.24)
MI	3.7	4.0	0.91 (0.70-1.18)
Stroke	1.3	1.1	1.22 (0.75-1.98)
PCI**	8.4	8.1	NS****
CABG***	12.7	12.8	NS****

* Patients with two or more events of different types appear more than once in columns but only once in rows.
**PCI = percutaneous intervention
***CABG = coronary artery bypass graft
****NS = non-significant; no detail on CI was reported for these items
‡ CVD: cardiovascular death includes cardiac death and fatal stroke. Sudden death is included in cardiac death.

In patients with an impaired left ventricular function (left ventricular ejection fraction LVEF <40%) total mortality and sudden death were higher and the impact of highly concentrated n-3 PUFA was more important in this subgroup of patients (Table 2).

Table 2. Mortality in subgroup of patients with impaired left ventricular function

Event	n-3 PUFAs	Control	RR (95% CI)
Total mortality	16.4	22.2	0.74 (0.48-0.97)
Sudden death	4.1	7.3	0.56 (0.29-1.03)

1.3. Cost Data

For the economic calculations of the model the cost of myocardial infarction (MI), ischaemic stroke, coronary artery bypass graft (CABG), percutaneous interventions (PCI) and cardiac death are to be applied (direct costs). Since the number of life-years gained is assessed lifelong also the costs during the extra years alive may be taken into account. We have done this for a secondary analysis (sensitivity analysis). Thereto, the average health expenditure per inhabitant in the target countries was searched (results are reported with and without this health expenditure in Table 4). On the website of the OECD, total expenditure per capita on health is reported for the 5 case countries (www.oecd.org). We doubled these costs (Table 3) to correct for the age and the history of disease (source: Belgian Federal Planning Office, 2003).

Australian cost data can be found on the national DRG website (http://www.health.gov.au/casemix/). The National Hospital Cost Data Collection (NHCDC) conducts an annual collection of hospital data from a sample of public and private acute care hospitals throughout Australia. The last data available at the moment of the model development were for the financial year 2001-2002. The increasing number of hospitals participating in the collection over the years provides increased robustness to the results and also helps to improve the methodology for data processing, analysis and reporting. The sample comprised 203 public hospitals and 83 private hospitals. The costs shown in Table 2 are based on a weighted average of the number of cases in private and public hospitals. (exchange rate Australian $ in 2002; 1 $A = € 0.60672).

Belgian costs were found in published literature. Muls *et al* reported on the cost of MI and stroke and Caro *et al* on the cost of CABG and PCI in Belgium [13],[14]. The costs of the year 1995 were updated to the year 2003 by using the mean Belgian health inflation rate from 1996-2002 (www.statgov.be). The cost of cardiovascular death was derived based on a patient chart review [15].

In a study by Grover *et al* on the cost-effectiveness of lipid-lowering with statins, the cost for acute hospitalisation of MI and stroke were reported for several countries including Canada [16]. The values from 2001 were updated to 2003 by using the Canadian specific medical inflation index (www.statcan.ca) (1 Euro = 1.6446 CAD May 2004).

The cost of acute events in Germany was provided based on official DRG (Diagnosis Related Groups) data (http://drg.uni-muenster.de/).

Calculating the cost of hospitalisations in Poland is complex. Until the end of the year 2003, 17 Regional Health Funds existed in Poland and each of them had own reimbursement politics. From January 1st 2004 on, one National Health Fund (NHF) was established and Regional Health Funds turned into Regional Divisions of the NHF with limited independence. So partial centralization of the system occurred in Poland in 2004 but there are still some differences in healthcare politics and reimbursement level in various parts of the country. Each procedure is valued for a number of points (worth of one point = 10 zlotys (current exchange rate: 1 Euro = 4.70 polish zlotys April 2004)). The value of one point for interventional procedures is the same for each region of the country. The exact amount of points depends on details of procedure performed by the service-provider. The costs needed were checked for 4 different regions of the country: Malopolska (Cracow), Wielkopolska (Warsaw region), Lublin (eastern part of Poland) as well as Katowice (Silesia region). The cost range obtained is shown in Table 3.

Table 3. Cost data used in the model

Cost item	Australia*		Belgium	Canada [16]		Germany**	Poland***	
	Au$	Euro	Euro	CAD	Euro	Euro	Cost (zloty)	Cost (€)
Non-fatal MI	3,248	1,971	9,822 [13]	8,099	4,925	3,123	7,123 - 7,678	1,515 - 1,634
Stroke	7,685	4,663	6,407	9,021	5,485	3,390	8,800 - 11,600	1,872 - 2,468
CABG	16,753	10,164	13,024 [14]	18,867	11,472	10,515	14,000	2,978
PTCA	5,302	3,217	5,502 [14]	8,292	5,042	3,004	7,076 - 7,869	1,505 - 1,674
Fatal MI	3,826	2,321	3,744 [15]	8,811	5,357	2,880	300	64
Sudden death	2,891	1,754	123 [15]	600	365	2,140	69	15
n-3 PUFA cost per day	1.40	0.85	1.25	1.16	0.74	1.04	5.07	1.08
Average cost per patient for the health care payer****	5,165	3,134	5,456	6,024	3,663	3,502	1,169	249

* http://www.health.gov.au/casemix/
** Official DRG: http://drg.uni-muenster.de/
*** National Health Fund
**** http://www.oecd.org

1.4. Life Expectancy

Life-years gained by highly concentrated n-3 PUFAs can be calculated, assuming that if an event is avoided this has long-term implications. Hence, the number of life-years that can be gained lifelong are taken into account.

Estimation of life expectancy after a cardiovascular event was evaluated by reviewing the literature and the Saskatchewan Health database [17]. The Saskatchewan database provides data that are quite recent (taking into account the needed follow-up time for such data) and based on a large population. Data were obtained from the Saskatchewan Health databases on patients with a diagnosis of MI occurring between 1985 and 1995 and with a follow-up updated to December 31, 2000 [17]. This database provides information on the life expectancy of patients with a MI who develop a new MI or a stroke.

The mean age of the patients included in the GISSI-Prevenzione study was 59.3 years [9]. Life expectancy results found in the Saskatchewan database for the age 62.5 years should be recalculated to the starting age and to the age of the second event in the GISSI-study. Indeed, the patients entered the model at the age of 59 years (GISSI-P study: 59.3 years) and it is assumed that the average event occurs after 1.75 years (see before). Thus, patients starting the model at an age of 59 years, will on average have their second event (MI or stroke) at age of 61 years. It is assumed that life expectancy after an event increases or decreases in function of age to the same extend as normal life expectancy. Based on the life expectancies in the different case countries in healthy people, life expectancies in the diseased population aged 61 was calculated (Table 4).

Thus, patients dying during the study period will lose about 13 life-years (life expectancy at study start 14.8 years minus time of average event, 1.75 years).

Table 4. Life expectancy after cardiovascular events in the different countries

Life expectancy at age 62.5 according Saskatchewan database [17]		
	LE (years)	**Sample size (n)**
First event		
Myocardial infarction	12.9	15,590
Further events in MI patients		
New MI	6.4	1,669
Ischaemic stroke	7.4	704

Recalculated life expectancy per country used in the model					
	Australia **LE** **(years)**	**Belgium** **LE** **(years)**	**Canada** **LE** **(years)**	**Germany** **LE** **(years)**	**Poland** **LE** **(years)**
First event					
Myocardial infarction	14.9	14.8	14.8	14.6	13.8
Further events in MI patients					
New MI	6.9	6.8	6.8	6.7	6.3
Ischaemic stroke	8.0	7.9	7.9	7.8	7.4

1.5. One Way Sensitivity Analyses

In the base-case it is assumed that if an event is avoided this also results in life-years gained after the 3.5-year study period, without taking into account costs that may be incurred during these additional life-years. As a sensitivity analysis it was taken into account that, if life-years gained are extrapolated lifelong that this also results in extra costs for the health care payer during these extra years of life (lifelong approach for life expectancy and costs). In another analysis it was assumed that only costs were made during the 3.5-year study period and that life-years were only gained during the 3.5-year study period and not extrapolated lifelong (truncation).

In the base-case it was assumed that the risk of sudden death with n-3 PUFAs was decreased from 7.2% to 5.1%, a relative reduction of 29.2%. Conversely, it can be said that mortality without n-3 PUFAs is relatively 41% higher as compared to treatment with n-3 PUFAs. In the sensitivity analysis the country specific effectiveness threshold for cost-effectiveness is searched, i.e. up to which level of effectiveness will the cost-effectiveness for n-3 PUFAs still be within societal willingness to pay limits. For Belgium and Germany no official willingness to pay level exists, so a tentative value of 20,000 Euro/LYG is used. In Poland, although not officially, a threshold of 10,640 Euro/LYG (50,000 zloty/LYG) is used. For Canada and Australia respectively 30,000 Euro/LYG and 47,000 Euro/LYG are used [18],[19].

Also, cost-effectiveness in the subgroup of patients with a history of MI and a decreased left ventricular ejection fraction was studied. It was anticipated that since these patients are at higher risk for sudden death, the value for money of n-3 PUFAs would be better in this subpopulation.

Finally, the impact of decreasing and increasing the cost of complications with 20% and discounting effects and costs with a range from 0 to 6% was evaluated.

1.6.   Monte Carlo Analysis

A 2nd order Monte Carlo simulation based on the 95% CIs obtained from the GISSI-Prevenzione study was performed (the model was run 1000 times) assuming a normal distribution for these clinical parameters. Whereas for four of the five countries studied the cost of complications was well-defined (official sources), for Poland there was more uncertainty around those costs (see before), therefore also the Polish costs were varied and this by using a triangular distribution with a minimum and maximum value.

1.7.   Budget Impact

Since resources are scarce it is of interest for the health care payer to know the budget impact of reimbursing given treatment strategies. An attempt was made to calculate the budget impact of reimbursing highly concentrated n-3 PUFAs in the 5 case countries. Therefore the number of patients eligible for treatment, thus the number of patients with an acute MI, was to be estimated.

Information on the number of MIs in Australia was found on an official website (www.aihw.gov.au/cvd/majordiseases/coronary.html). In 2001-2002, there were 159,561 hospitalisations for coronary heart disease. Of the hospitalisations for coronary heart disease, angina accounted for over half (87,023) and AMI for around one-quarter (40,333).

For Belgium, data on the number of patients being hospitalized with an MI can be retrieved on the following governmental website: https://tct.fgov.be/. Latest data available are from 2001. The sum of the numbers of hospitalizations mentioned under the APR-DRG 174 (percutaneous cardiovascular interventions with MI) and 190 (circulatory disease with MI) results in a total number of eligible patients of 13,608.

Information on the incidence of myocardial infarction in Canada is provided by the Heart and Stroke Foundation Canada in its report "The changing face of heart disease and stroke in Canada 2000" (http://www.phac-aspc.gc.ca/ccdpc-cpcmc/cvd-mcv/publications/pdf/card2ke.pdf).

In this report it is estimated that in the year 2003 and 40,000 men and 22,500 women were hospitalized for an acute MI of which 12.1% died during the first month (http://www.statcan.ca). Thus, about 55,000 patients are eligible for treatment with n-3 PUFAs each year.

In Germany detail on the number of hospitalisation with MI can be found on the website www.gbe-bund.de. According this website there are about 130,000 patients having an MI each year. All the patients hospitalized (thus, reaching the hospital alive) are eligible for treatment.

There is no epidemiological study derived information on the number of myocardial infarctions in Poland. But different sources mention a number between 80,000 and 100,000 MI per year [20]. The number of acute coronary syndromes was estimated to be about 240,000 (Guidelines of Polish Cardiac Society).

No data on pre-hospital mortality for the whole population of Poland is available. An epidemiological study performed for population of middle and eastern Poland is most country specific source of information available for Polish population. Of all subjects comprised in the study 23.9% died during pre-hospital period. The pre-hospital mortality due to acute MI was significantly higher in men (26%) compared to women (17%) [21]. The Pol-MONICA study revealed data concerning pre-hospital death in the population of Warsaw which amounted to 28% [22].

The % of patients surviving the first 30 days after MI with ST elevation is about 8.4% (extrapolation of the Euro Heart Survey of acute coronary syndromes) [23].

This means that between 55,766 and 69,708 patients with MI could be eligible for treatment with highly concentrated n-3 PUFA (80,000 or 100,000 - 23.9% dying before hospital - 8.4% dying in the first month after MI).

2.   Results

2.1.   Base-Case

Treatment with highly concentrated n-3 PUFAs yielded between 0.260 (Poland) and 0.284 (Australia) life-years, at an additional cost of € 807 (Canada) to € 1,451 (Belgium) (Table 5). The incremental cost-effectiveness ratio (ICER) varied between € 2,867 (Canada) and € 5,154 (Belgium) per LYG.

Table 5. Cost (€) and effectiveness (LYG) results

Strategy	Base-case					Lifelong costs and life expectancy*			Truncation at 3.5 years[§]		
	Cost	Incr Cost	LY	LYG	Incr C/LYG	Cost	Incr Cost	Incr C/LYG	LY	LYG	Incr C/LYG
Australia											
No n-3 PUFA	1,709		12.569			26,771			3.157		
n-3 PUFA	2,681	973	12.852	0.284	3,429	28,402	1,631	5,750	3.193	0.037	26,528
Belgium											
No n-3 PUFA	2,747		12.486			50,447			3.157		
n-3 PUFA	4,198	1,451	12.767	0.281	5,154	53,150	2,704	9,606	3.193	0.037	39,568
Canada											
No n-3 PUFA	2,190		12.486			32,844			3.157		
n-3 PUFA	2,997	807	12.767	0.281	2,867	34,457	1,612	5,728	3.193	0.037	22,008
Germany											
No n-3 PUFA	1,798		12.32			31,866			3.157		
n-3 PUFA	2,982	1,185	12.598	0.277	4,274	33,841	1,975	7,124	3.193	0.037	32,308
Poland											
No n-3 PUFA	559		11.659			3,200			3.157		
n-3 PUFA	1,821	1,263	11.919	0.260	4,856	4,532	1,332	5,123	3.193	0.037	34,441

* Life-years gained are the same as in the base-case.
[§] Costs are the same as in the base-case.

2.2.   One Way Sensitivity Analyses

If the lifelong approach on life expectancy and costs is taken total costs are considerably increased (more than tenfold), and the ICER almost doubles. If the truncated approach is used (costs and life-years gained cut at 3.5 years) the ICER increases importantly (almost factor 8) (see Table 5).

Decreasing and increasing the cost of complications (MI, stroke, sudden death, CABG and PCI) with 20% changes the ICER relatively with less than 1%.

Varying the discount rate on costs and effects between 0 and 6% results in a 6% change in ICER.

Although total cost increases in the subpopulation of patients with impaired left ventricular function, ICER of n-3 PUFA compared to no treatment decreases to about 1,500 Euro/LYG in the 5 countries studied, due to a more than doubling in the number of life-years gained.

Before the country specific willingness to pay is reached, the risk of sudden death under treatment with n-3 PUFAs can be 40%, 33%, 38%, 34% and 24% higher compared to baseline (5.1%) for respectively Australia, Belgium, Canada, Germany and Poland (example of Poland the willingness to pay threshold is 10,640 Euro/LYG. If the risk of sudden death is 24% higher compared to the 5.1% baseline (= 6.32%) the calculated ICER becomes 10,500 Euro/LYG, see Figure 2).

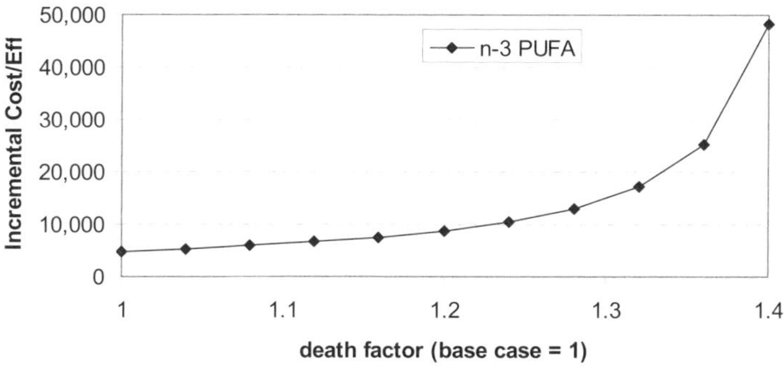

Figure 2. Impact of risk of sudden death with n-3 PUFA on ICER (Polish example).

2.3.   Monte Carlo Analysis

Based on the 2nd order Monte Carlo simulation using the 95% CIs obtained from the GISSI-Prevenzione study, the cost-effectiveness acceptability curves for the different countries were drawn. From a willingness to pay of 20,000 Euro/LYG on, administering highly concentrated n-3 PUFAs is cost-effective in more than 99% of the simulations in the five countries (see Figure 3).

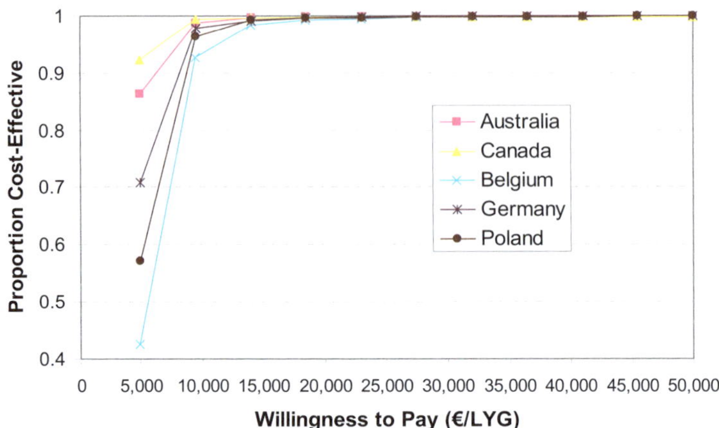

Figure 3. Acceptability curves.

2.4.   *Budget Impact Analysis*

A 3-year budget forecast is calculated for the 5 countries. Each year the same number (country dependent) of patients are added for treatment. It is assumed that all eligible patients are treated with highly concentrated n-3 PUFAs. It is assumed that events are equally distributed over time in the GISSI-Prevenzione study. This assumption is supported by a report of Marchioli *et al* [24]. The average yearly drug cost for highly concentrated n-3 PUFA per patient, taking into account mortality, was calculated to be 990 Euro, 1,457 Euro, 822 Euro, 1,217 Euro and 1,257 Euro for respectively Australia, Belgium, Canada, Germany and Poland. These costs are used to calculate the annual and 3-year budget impact.

In Table 6 the budget impact in the different countries is shown. In the second column the cost of treating the patients with n-3 PUFAs is shown, whereas in the third and fourth column it is shown what is the total cost of patients with an MI not treated (third column) and treated with n-3 PUFAs (fourth column). The impact on the total budget will be highest in Poland.

Table 6. 3-year budget impact based on the number of patients eligible for treatment with n-3 PUFAs in the different countries

Year	Drug cost (n-3 PUFA)	Health care budget for population with recent MI	
		No treatment	Treated with n-3 PUFA
Australia	N = 40,333		
1	11,408,477*	19,694,028[§]	30,895,078
2	22,816,954	39,388,055	61,790,156
3	34,225,431	59,082,083	92,685,234
Total	**68,450,863**	**118,164,166**	**185,370,468**
Belgium	N = 13,600		
1	5,661,486	8,731,200	16,312,229
2	11,322,971	17,462,400	32,624,457
3	16,984,457	26,193,600	48,936,686
Total	**33,968,914**	**52,387,200**	**97,873,371**
Canada	N = 55,000		
1	12,917,143	34,414,286	47,095,714
2	25,834,286	68,828,571	94,191,429
3	38,751,429	103,242,857	141,287,143
Total	**77,502,857**	**206,485,714**	**282,574,286**
Germany	N = 133,000		
1	46,246,000	68,324,000	113,316,000
2	92,492,000	136,648,000	226,632,000
3	138,738,000	204,972,000	339,948,000
Total	**277,476,000**	**409,944,000**	**679,896,000**
Poland	N = 60,000		
1	21,548,571	9,582,857	31,217,143
2	43,097,143	19,165,714	62,434,286
3	64,645,714	28,748,571	93,651,429
Total	**129,291,429**	**57,497,143**	**187,302,857**

*The yearly drug cost per patients is € 283 (€ 990/3.5-year study period). This € 283 is multiplied with 40,333 patients = € 11,408,407. The second and the third year another 40,333 patients are added. The average drug cost is an outcome of the model and already corrects for patients dying during the study period.

[§]No treatment costs € 1,709 over the 3.5-year study period (see Table 5). Thus the average cost per year is € 1,709/3.5 = € 488, multiplied with 40,333 = 19,6940,028.

3.   Discussion

In the health-economic analysis presented here the use of highly concentrated n-3 PUFAs in the secondary prevention after MI appears to be a cost-effective alternative for the five countries studied. Incremental cost-effectiveness ratio varied between € 2,867 (Canada) and € 5,154 (Belgium). Sensitivity analyses have shown the robustness of the results.

Especially in patients with a history of MI and an impaired left ventricular function, patients known to be at an even higher risk of sudden death, treatment with highly concentrated n-3 PUFAs appears to be of large interest.

One could argue that the population included in the GISSI-Prevenzione study is not comparable with the population of the five case countries since the study was performed in Italy, a country with another (lower) risk of cardiovascular disease. Abhyankar [25] compared the effectiveness of n-3 PUFAs with the effectiveness of statins in large secondary prevention trials and concluded that the study results fit in well with the other studies performed in secondary prevention and that the studied population in the GISSI-Prevenzione study is comparable to the population included in the other secondary prevention studies [24]. Also, the lipid levels of the patients included in the GISSI-Prevenzione study are only slightly higher compared to the European population [26].

It should be noted that the GISSI-Prevenzione study was conducted between October 1993-September 1995, at a moment when for example statins were not yet recommended in the secondary prevention after MI. Use of statins increased from approximately 4.7% at baseline to approximately 45% at the end of the study, but the proportion of patients using these drugs in each study group was similar throughout the study. There were no differences on the relative risk for all-cause mortality found between treatment groups receiving highly concentrated n-3 PUFAs with or without concomitant use of statins, making the positive effect seen clearly attributable to the use of n-3 PUFAs in these MI patients.

Since only one controlled clinical trial was used to populate the model, not many assumptions were to be made to calculate cost-effectiveness.

We realistically assumed that if an event is avoided, a number of life-years can be gained. Indeed, epidemiological surveys have shown that life expectancy is lower after 2 MIs than after 1 MI (Saskatchewan database) [17]. Several authors applied this approach to assess life expectancy [27],[28],[29]. Using the lifelong approach results in a very cost-effective strategy in the 5 case countries.

In their health-economic evaluation Franzosi *et al* estimated that if a patient did not die during the study period he gained life-years until the end of the study period, which was 3.5 years [12]. In their analysis applied to the Italian population, the ICER for highly concentrated n-3 PUFAs in the base-case scenario was 24,603 Euro (1999 values) per life-year gained (95% confidence interval: 22,646 to 26,930). If we would consider the same approach, thus considering only the 3.5-year study period, ICER's are in the same range as the value of Franzosi *et al*, and administering n-3 PUFAs is within the range of what is accepted as cost-effectiveness in Australia and Canada.

Compared to other reimbursed treatments in the secondary prevention after myocardial infarction highly concentrated n-3 PUFAs seem at least as cost-effective as, for example, cholesterol-lowering therapy with statins in secondary prevention of coronary artery disease or other secondary prevention means [13]. Brown *et al* showed that the cost-effectiveness of eptifibatide, a glycoproteine IIb/IIIa inhibitor in patients with unstable angina and myocardial infarction (based on the PURSUIT trial) ranged from € 9,603 to € 18,115/LYG in Europe [30]. Based on the results of the CAPRIE trial, Haldeman *et al* calculated the cost-effectiveness of clopidogrel in secondary prevention in the Swiss setting. The cost per life-year saved found was € 14,850 [31].

The budget impact analysis show that, due to the important number of patients that are eligible for treatment with n-3 PUFAs, the impact on the health care payers budget can be considerable.

We therefore conclude that administering highly concentrated n-3 PUFAs is cost-effective in the secondary prevention of cardiovascular disease after MI. For budgetary reasons, a limitation to patients with a history of MI and an impaired left ventricular function may be envisaged, but purely based on cost-effectiveness this limitation to the highest risk group does not seem to be justifiable, since the cost-effectiveness in the larger group post-MI is very good as well, with a high cost-effectiveness acceptability curve.

Acknowledgement

This study was carried out by HEDM-IMS under a grant from Solvay Pharmaceuticals GmbH. The study was performed independently by HEDM-IMS, and the manuscript was approved by each author before submission. Solvay had the opportunity to comment on a draft of the manuscript and the authors were free to decline publication.

References

[1]   E. Braunwald. Evolution of the management of acute myocardial infarction: a 20th century saga. *Lancet* **352** (1998) 1771-1774.

[2]   S. Capewell, B.M. Livingston, K. MacIntyre *et al.* Trends in case-fatality in 117 718 patients admitted with acute myocardial infarction in Scotland. *Eur. Heart J.* **21** (2000) 1833-1840.

[3]   S.M. Haffner, S. Lehto, T. Rönnemaa *et al.* Mortality from coronary heart disease in subjects with type 2 diabetes and in nondiabetic subjects with and without prior myocardial infarction. *N. Engl. J. Med.* **339** (1998) 229-234.

[4]   F.C. Lampe, P.H. Whincup, S.G. Wannamethee *et al.* The natural history of prevalent ischaemic heart disease in middle-aged men. *Eur. Heart J.* **21** (2000) 1052-1062.

[5]   M. de Lorgeril and P. Salen. Diet as preventive medicine in cardiology. *Curr. Opin. Cardiol.* **15** (2000) 364-370.

[6]   H.V. Huikuri, A. Castellanos, R.J. Myerburg. Sudden death due to cardiac arrhythmias. *N. Engl. J. Med.* **345** (2001) 1473-1482.

[7]   R.J. Myerburg and P.M. Spooner. Opportunities for sudden death prevention: directions for new clinical and basic research. *Cardiovasc. Res.* **50** (2001) 177-185.

[8]   S.G. Priori, E. Aliot, C. Blomstrom-Lundqvist *et al.* Task force on sudden cardiac death of the European Society of Cardiology. *Eur. Heart J.* **22** (2001) 1374-1450.

[9]   GISSI-Prevenzione Investigators. Dietary supplementation with n-3 polyunsaturated fatty acids and vitamin E after myocardial infraction: results of the GISSI-Prevenzione trial. Gruppo Italiano per lo Studio della Sopravvivenza nell'Infarto miocardico. *Lancet* **354** (1999) 447-455.

[10]   M. Johannesson, D. Meltzer, R.M. O'Conor. Incorporating future costs in medical cost-effectiveness analysis: implications for the cost-effectiveness of the treatment of hypertension. *Med. Decis. Making* **17** (1997) 382-389.

[11]   R. Marchioli. Treatment with n-3 polyunsaterated fatty acids after myocardial infarction: results of the GISSI-Prevenzione Trial. *Eur. Heart J. Suppl.* **3** (2001) D85-D97.

[12]   M.G. Franzosi, M. Brunetti, R. Marchioli *et al.* Cost-effectiveness analysis of n-3 polyunsaturated fatty acids (PUFA) after myocardial infarction: results from Gruppo Italiano per lo Studio della Sopravvivenza nell'Infarto (GISSI)-Prevenzione Trial. *Pharmacoeconomics* **19** (2001) 411-420.

[13]   E. Muls, E. Van Ganse, M.C. Closon. Cost-effectiveness of pravastatin in secondary prevention of coronary heart disease: comparison between Belgium and the United States of a projected risk model. *Atherosclerosis* **137 (Suppl.)** (1998) S111-S116.

[14]   J.J. Caro, K.F. Huybrechts, G. De Backer *et al.* Are the WOSCOPS clinical and economic findings generalizable to other populations? A case study for Belgium. *Acta Cardiol.* **55** (2000) 239-246.

[15]   M. Lamotte, K. Caekelbergh, L. Annemans *et al.* Assessment of the cost of cardiovascular death. *Value in Health* **6** (2003) 658.

[16]   S.A. Grover, L. Coupal, H. Zowall *et al.* How cost-effective is the treatment of dyslipidemia in patients with diabetes but without cardiovascular disease? *Diabetes Care* **24** (2001) 45-50.

[17]   L. Annemans, M. Lamotte, E. Levy *et al.* Cost-effectiveness analysis of clopidogrel versus aspirin in patients with atherothrombosis based on the CAPRIE trial. *JME* **6** (2003) 55-68.

[18]   P. Coy, J. Schaafsma, J.A. Schofield. The cost-effectiveness and cost-utility of high-dose palliative radiotherapy for advanced non-small-cell lung cancer. *Int. J. Radiat. Oncol. Biol. Phys.* **48** (2000) 1025-1033.

[19]   J.A. Mauskopf, S.C. Cates, A.D. Griffin *et al.* Cost effectiveness of zanamivir for the treatment of influenza in a high risk population in Australia. *Pharmacoeconomics* **17** (2000) 611-620.

[20]   G. Opolski, K.J. Filipiak, L. Poloński. *Ostre zespoły wieńcowe.* Urban & Partner (2002) 8-11.

[21]   W. Witczak and S. Tokarski. Pre-hospital mortality due to myocardial infarction in the population of middle-eastern Poland. *Med. Sci. Monit.* **5** (1999) 1163-1167.

[22]   A. Pająk, K. Jamrozik, E. Kawalec. Myocardial infarction--risks and procedures. Longitudinal observation of a population of 280,000 women and men--Project POL-MONI CA Krakow. III: Epidemiology and treatment of myocardial infarction. *Przegl. Lek.* **53** (1996) 767-778 (*in Polish*).

[23]   D. Hasdai, S. Behar, L. Wallentin. A prospective survey of the characteristics, treatments and outcomes of patients with acute coronary syndromes in Europe and the Mediterranean basin: the Euro Heart Survey of Acute Coronary Syndromes (Euro Heart Survey ACS). *Eur. Heart J.* **23** (2002) 1190-1201.

[24]   R. Marchioli, F. Barzi, E. Bomba *et al.* Early protection against sudden death by n-3 polyunsaturated fatty acids after myocardial infarction: time-course analysis of the results of the Gruppo Italiano per lo Studio della Sopravvivenza nell'Infarto Miocardico (GISSI)-Prevenzione. *Circulation* **105** (2002) 1897-1903.

[25]   B. Abhyankar. Further reduction in mortality following myocardial infarction. *Hosp. Med.* **63** (2002) 610-614.

[26]   EUROASPIRE II Study Group. Lifestyle and risk factor management and use of drug therapies in coronary patients from 15 countries: principal results from EUROASPIRE II Euro Heart Survey Programme. *Eur. Heart J.* **22** (2001) 554-572.

[27]   J. Caro, W. Klittich, A. McGuire *et al.* The West of Scotland coronary prevention study: economic benefit analysis of primary prevention with pravastatin. *BMJ* **315** (1997) 1577-1582.

[28]   P.D. Pharoah and W. Hollingworth. Cost effectiveness of lowering cholesterol concentration with statins in patients with and without pre-existing coronary heart disease: life table method applied to health authority population. *BMJ* **312** (1996) 1443-1448.

[29]   J. Tsevat, K.M. Kuntz, E.J. Orav *et al.* Cost-effectiveness of pravastatin therapy for survivors of myocardial infarction with average cholesterol levels. *Am. Heart J.* **141** (2001) 727-734.

[30]   R.E. Brown, R.A. Henderson, D. Koster *et al.* Cost effectiveness of eptifibatide in acute coronary syndromes; an economic analysis of Western European patients enrolled in the PURSUIT trial. The Platelet IIa/IIb in unstable Angina: Receptor Suppression Using Integrilin Therapy. *Eur. Heart J.* **23** (2002) 50-58.

[31]   R. Haldemann, T.F. Luscher, T.D. Szucs. Cost effectiveness of clopidogrel in secondary cardiovascular prevention: a cost-effectiveness analysis based on the Caprie Study. *Schweiz Rundsch. Med. Prax.* **90** (2001) 539-545 (*in German*).

OMACOR® in Clinical Development: A Survey of Current Trials

Hogne Vik
Pronova Biocare, P.O. Box 420, N-1327 Lysaker, Norway

Abstract. OMACOR® is the focus of an extensive and ambitious clinical development program that seeks to build on the results of the Gruppo Italiano per lo Studio della Sopravvivenza nell'Infarto Miocardico (GISSI)-Prevenzione study. Studies currently in progress include very large clinical outcome trials designed to evaluate the impact of OMACOR® on death and major morbid events in defined patient populations such as individuals with heart failure or diabetes, specialist investigations in very high-risk populations such as patients requiring hemodialysis, and a range of specialized studies concerned with mechanisms of action and effects on biochemical and laboratory indices. The emergence of results from these studies can be expected to define a spectrum of indications for OMACOR® in the management of cardiovascular and renal disease.

Keywords: Highly purified omega-3 polyunsaturated fatty acids, OMACOR®, randomized controlled trials, cardiovascular disease, diabetes, hypertriglyceridemia, IgA nephropathy

1. Introduction

Evidence-based medicine (EBM) has acknowledged roots in the 19th century but the term as currently applied and understood (or sometimes misunderstood!) refers to a style of medical enquiry that is little more than 10 years old [1]. Despite its relative novelty, EBM has advanced rapidly, and in many regions of the world and arenas of medicine is now established as a central feature of clinical research and an essential requirement in the development of rational best clinical practice. Numerous specialist centers dedicated to the practice of EBM have been established (notably the Cochrane Collaboration), as well as a variety of journal and online resources.

The stated objectives of modern-day EBM, as summarized by one of its proponents, are "the conscientious, explicit and judicious use of current best evidence in making decisions about the care of individual patients" [2]. These principles place a premium on the quality of evidence used to guide clinical decision making; the current hierarchy of evidence assigns special importance to meta-analyses of randomized controlled trials (RCTs) [3]. It will at once be apparent, however, that good-quality RCTs themselves are a prerequisite for any useful meta-analysis. The development and conduct of robust RCTs is thus central to the practice of EBM; even a brief survey of this area must register the significance of Archibald Cochrane's pioneering work and inspiration [4].

The science of clinical trial design has evolved rapidly in the modern era of EBM. Issues currently under discussion include the role and relevance of placebo [5], the potential for 'n-of-1' RCTs [6], and the possibility of undertaking studies via the Internet [7]. At the same time, the status of EBM and RCTs - or perhaps more exactly the status and influence attached to the results of such trials when trying to integrate EBM into routine clinical practice - is a source of energetic and thoughtful debate [8-11]. It may be argued, for example, that the restrictive terms necessary to conduct properly 'controlled' trials can sometimes lead to an overly narrow stratum of patients being enrolled. This, in turn, may create difficulties in the interpretation of the results of such studies and their application to a wider candidate population: the studies are said to lack 'generalizability' [12,13]. Such criticisms notwithstanding, it remains the case that properly conducted RCTs, which eliminate sources of bias and other possible extraneous influences, provide the best means currently available for the evaluation of new therapeutic ideas. To that extent (and without being regarded as infallible or incapable of improvement) RCTs serve the requirement to use 'current best evidence' in EBM and have considerably aided the development of many current-day therapeutic principles.

RCTs have also served the equally valuable purpose of establishing that certain interventions expected to be clinically beneficial are, in fact, not. Examples of this include hormone replacement therapy (HRT), vitamin E supplements, and homocysteine-lowering interventions, all of which have been advocated for the prevention of cardiovascular disease (CVD) on the basis of epidemiological and experimental observations.

Advocates of vitamin E had argued that the correlation between (at least relative) vitamin insufficiency and increased risk for CVD intimated a role for vitamin E supplements in the reduction of cardiovascular risk. However, RCTs such as Gruppo Italiano per lo Studio della Sopravvivenza nell'Infarto Miocardico (GISSI)-Prevenzione [14], Heart Outcomes Prevention Evaluation (HOPE) [15], the UK Medical Research Council Heart Protection Study [16], and the US Women's Health Study [17] revealed no benefit from such supplements, in either primary or secondary prevention. (It may be remarked in passing, however, that one response to the demonstration that vitamin E in the form of alpha-tocopherol does not reduce cardiovascular risk has been to suggest that benefit may be derived from the gamma-tocopherol form [18]. This reaction illustrates how RCTs may stimulate further research ideas while simultaneously revealing that the power of RCTs to provide a 'definitive' answer to an issue is sometimes exaggerated.)

The Nordic Vitamin Trial (NORVIT) has recently produced no evidence that treatment with 40 mg/day of vitamin B6 or 0.8 mg/day of folic acid for 3 years reduced cardiovascular risk in post-myocardial infarction (MI) patients despite producing substantial reductions ($\approx$30%) in plasma homocysteine levels. Indeed, cardiovascular risk, which was unchanged in patients randomized to either supplement, increased by 20% in patients given both [19]. These data confound the belief, developed from epidemiological data, that lowering plasma homocysteine may reduce cardiovascular risk. The lack of effect of folic acid, regarded as the preferred intervention for lowering homocysteine [20], may well signal the beginning of the end for this line of research, at least with regard to secondary CVD prevention. A total of 12 studies of homocysteine-lowering interventions are in progress and a meta-analysis of these studies (n$\approx$32,000) is planned, to provide a 'best-evidence' perspective of this issue [21].

OMACOR® was shown to be highly effective as an adjunct to usual care in the secondary prevention of major cardiovascular events in the same GISSI-Prevenzione study that found no benefit from vitamin E. In accordance with the principles and spirit of EBM, OMACOR® is now being evaluated in an extensive clinical trials program designed to investigate whether it has clinical applications additional to those confirmed in GISSI-Prevenzione.

These studies may be classified as trials of OMACOR® at daily doses (e.g. 1-2 g/day) similar to that used in GISSI-Prevenzione (1 g/day) and studies of higher doses, such as have previously been used in the management of hypertriglyceridemia.

2. Ongoing Controlled Trials of OMACOR® 1-2 g/day

2.1. ASCEND: A Study of Cardiovascular Events in Diabetes

2.1.1. Rationale

- Diabetes affects about 150 million individuals worldwide. Moreover, the prevalence is increasing rapidly, and it is estimated that there will be 300 million people worldwide with type-2 diabetes mellitus by 2025, and a further 30 million with type-1 disease [22].
- There is consistent evidence from observational studies that consumption of omega-3 polyunsaturated fatty acids (PUFAs) is associated with lower rates of CVD (particularly cardiac and sudden death). Use of highly purified omega-3 PUFAs in MI survivors has been associated with improved clinical prognosis [14]. To date, however, no large-scale trials have examined the potential of omega-3 PUFAs for preventing vascular events in people with diabetes who do not have diagnosed arterial disease.
- The value of aspirin in the secondary prevention of heart attacks and strokes has been amply demonstrated for many categories of high-risk patients with diagnosed arterial disease, whether or not they have diabetes. However, many young and middle-aged people with diabetes are still at significant risk for CVD even when they do not have manifest arterial disease, and there is still substantial uncertainty about the role of aspirin for the prevention of heart attacks and strokes among apparently healthy people with diabetes.

2.1.2. Objective

- To determine whether OMACOR® (1 g/day) and/or aspirin 100 mg/day, when added to existing standard therapy, can prevent cardiovascular events in patients who have diabetes but do not have clinically manifest arterial disease at baseline.

2.1.3. Design (Table 1)

- Randomized, placebo-controlled, double-blind, 2×2 factorial, multicenter study.
- Patients receive OMACOR® or aspirin, or OMACOR® plus aspirin, or double placebo in addition to standard therapy.

Table 1. Design of ASCEND

	Subgroup A: Aspirin arm **(n = 5000)**	**Subgroup B: Placebo arm** **(n = 5000)**
Subgroup 1: omega-3 PUFA arm (n = 5000)	Aspirin 100 mg/day + omega-3 PUFAs 1 g/day (n = 2500)	Aspirin placebo + omega-3 PUFAs 1 g/day (n = 2500)
Subgroup 2: placebo arm (n = 5000)	Aspirin 100 mg/day + omega-3 PUFA placebo (n = 2500)	Double placebo (n = 2500)

2.1.4. Study Medication Dosages

- 1 g/day OMACOR®.
- 100 mg/day aspirin (1 tablet).
- Matching double placebos.

2.1.5. Planned Sample Size

- 2500 patients per arm; total number of patients: 10,000.

2.1.6. Patients/Participation Criteria

- Men or women aged >40 years with diabetes (type-1 or 2).
- No history of overt vascular disease at baseline.
- No clear indication for aspirin.
- No contraindications to the use of aspirin.
- No evident life-threatening conditions (e.g. cancer).

2.1.7. Exclusion Criteria

- Confirmed prior MI, stroke or transient ischemic attack (TIA) or coronary or non-coronary revascularization.
- Currently using anticoagulants including, but not limited to, aspirin or warfarin.

2.1.8. Planned Duration of Follow-up

- Mean 5 years.

2.1.9. Primary End-Points

- Intention-to-treat comparison of the effects of omega-3 PUFAs 1 g/day vs. placebo on the overall incidence of serious vascular events, defined as: non-fatal MI, non-fatal stroke or vascular death, excluding confirmed cerebral hemorrhage (i.e. event rate in Subgroup 1 vs. event rate in Subgroup 2 in Table 1).
- Intention-to-treat comparison of the effects of aspirin vs. placebo on the overall incidence of serious vascular events, defined as: non-fatal MI, non-fatal stroke or vascular death, excluding confirmed cerebral hemorrhage (i.e. event rate in Subgroup A vs. event rate in Subgroup B in Table 1).

2.1.10. Secondary End-Points

The principal subsidiary comparisons will be of the effect of OMACOR® or aspirin vs. placebo on:
- The incidence of serious vascular events, and the combined end-point of serious vascular events or coronary or non-coronary revascularization in various prognostic subgroups (e.g. older vs. younger, men vs. women, longer- vs. shorter-duration diabetes); and in the presence and absence of the other study treatments.

- The incidence of confirmed cerebral hemorrhage and, separately, of other 'major hemorrhage' (defined as any other bleeding episode that requires hospitalization or transfusion, or that is fatal or disabling).

2.1.11. Tertiary End-Points

Comparison of the effects of study medication vs. placebo on:
- Total and cause-specific mortality.
- Total coronary events, i.e. non-fatal MI, coronary death or coronary revascularizations, i.e. coronary artery bypass graft (CABG) and percutaneous transluminal coronary angioplasty (PTCA).
- Non-hemorrhagic strokes.
- Venous thromboembolism.
- Total and site-specific cancers.
- Hospitalizations for various other causes.

2.1.12. Other

- The study is being supported by the British Heart Foundation.

2.1.13. Schedule

- Study start: March 2005.
- Recruitment of patients: ongoing.
- Anticipated completion date: March 2011.

ClinicalTrials.gov Identifier: NCT00135226.
ISRCTN Identifier: 60635500.

2.2. AFORRD: Atorvastatin in Factorial with Omega-3 Fatty Acid Risk Reduction in Patients with Type-2 Diabetes

2.2.1. Rationale

- People with type-2 diabetes mellitus are at markedly greater risk for coronary heart disease (CHD) than the general population. Statin therapy to lower low-density lipoprotein (LDL) cholesterol has been shown to substantially reduce CHD risk in people with type-2 diabetes [23].
- However, it remains uncertain (a) whether all patients with type-2 diabetes need statin therapy and (b) whether a fixed dose of statin can be used successfully in all cases. Moreover, some patients may require additional therapy to regulate triglycerides. This might be achieved by combining a fibrate with statin therapy but this confers a small but tangible risk of myositis or rhabdomyolysis.
- Omega-3 PUFAs 2-4 g/day have been shown to lower triglyceride levels in patients with hypertriglyceridemia and, at a lower dose of 1 g/day, to reduce mortality in post-MI patients [20,30]. The tolerability profile of omega-3 PUFAs is considered highly satisfactory. Hence, omega-3 PUFAs may be an effective and acceptable option for use in combination with a statin.

2.2.2. Objectives

To answer the following questions:
- What proportion of type-2 diabetes patients managed in primary care are candidates for LDL cholesterol-lowering therapy?
- In what proportion of candidate patients will a fixed 20 mg/day dose of atorvastatin reduce the estimated 10-year CHD risk to <15%?
- What is the effect of doubling the atorvastatin dose to 40 mg/day in patients whose estimated 10-year CHD risk remains >15% at 20 mg/day?
- What is the effect of a 2 g/day fixed dose of omega-3 PUFAs on triglyceride levels in patients treated/not treated with a statin?
- Can adherence to study medication be improved by the introduction of simple techniques in general practice?

2.2.3. Design (Table 2)

- Randomized, double-blind, 2×2 factorial, multicenter study.
- Patients are randomized to omega-3 PUFAs or atorvastatin, or both, or matching placebo/comparators.

Table 2. Design of AFORRD

	Atorvastatin arm (n = 500)	**Placebo arm (n = 500)**
Omega-3 PUFA arm (n = 500)	Atorvastatin 20 mg/day* + omega-3 PUFAs 2 g/day (n = 250)	Atorvastatin placebo + omega-3 PUFAs 2 g/day (n = 250)
Placebo arm (n = 500)	Atorvastatin 20 mg/day* + olive oil (omega-3 PUFA control) (n = 250)	Atorvastatin placebo + olive oil (omega-3 PUFA control) (n = 250)

*Dose doubled to 40 mg/day if LDL cholesterol levels ≥2.6 mmol/L after 16 weeks.

2.2.4. Study Medication Dosages

- 2 g/day OMACOR®.
- 20 or 40 mg/day atorvastatin.
- Matching placebos.

2.2.5. Patients/Participation Criteria

- Aged >18 years with type-2 diabetes diagnosed for ≥3 months.
- No known CHD.
- Not taking prescribed lipid-lowering therapy.
- Triglycerides <8.0 mmol/L.

2.2.6. Planned Sample Size

- 250 patients per arm; total number of patients: 1,000.

2.2.7. Methods

- Patients from 70 UK practices have been randomized in a 2×2 factorial design comparing OMACOR® with olive oil and, simultaneously, a fixed dose of atorvastatin (20 mg/day) with placebo. Ten-year CHD risk will be estimated using the UK Prospective Diabetes Study Risk Engine© at entry, and at 16 and 52 weeks. Atorvastatin dosage will be doubled to 40 mg/day (with equivalent placebo in the control group) in patients whose estimated CHD risk remains >15% at 16 weeks.
- A range of patient-centered techniques intended to improve adherence to medication will be deployed at half of the participating centers. At all sites, compliance with study medication will be monitored by the use of 'smart' containers that record the time and date of use.

2.2.8. Planned Duration of Follow-Up

- 52 weeks.

2.2.9. Primary End-Points

- Proportion of patients treated with omega-3 PUFAs 2 g/day that have triglyceride levels of <1.5 mmol/L at 16 weeks.
- Proportion of patients treated with atorvastatin 20 mg/day that have LDL cholesterol levels of <2.6 mmol/L at 16 weeks.

2.2.10. Secondary End-Points

- Proportion of patients treated with omega-3 PUFAs 2 g/day that have triglyceride levels of <1.5 mmol/L at 52 weeks.
- Proportion of patients treated with atorvastatin 20 mg/day that have LDL cholesterol levels of <2.6 mmol/L at 52 weeks.
- Proportion of patients with an estimated 10-year CHD risk of <15% at 16 and 52 weeks.
- Effect of behavioral intervention on adherence with study medication.
- Health-economic evaluation of predicted treatment effects on CHD rates.

2.2.11. Laboratory Measurements

- Lipid profiles.

2.2.12. Schedule

- Randomization completed July 2005; 800 randomized.
- Results anticipated: late 2006.

ClinicalTrials.gov Identifier: NCT00141232.
ISRCTN Identifier: 76737502.

2.3. ORIGIN: Outcome Reduction with Initial Glargine Intervention

2.3.1. Rationale

- Diabetes and dysglycemia are independently associated with cardiovascular events such as MI and stroke. Both the population prevalence of diabetes and the number of cases are expected to approximately double between 2000 and 2030, by which time more than 300 million people are expected to have the disease [25]. Moreover, there is persuasive evidence that the risk for vascular complications associated with type-2 diabetes may extend to individuals with glucose abnormalities who do not meet the criteria for frank diabetes. As many as two-thirds of people who experience a heart attack have impaired fasting glucose (IFG), impaired glucose tolerance (IGT), and/or early type-2 diabetes.
- Highly purified omega-3 PUFAs, given at low dose (1 g/day), have been shown to reduce mortality in post-MI patients with or without diabetes [14].

2.3.2. Objectives

- To determine whether highly purified omega-3 PUFAs can reduce cardiovascular mortality in people with IFG, IGT, or early diabetes, compared with placebo.
- To determine whether glargine-mediated normoglycemia, compared with standard diabetes care, can reduce cardiovascular morbidity and/or mortality in people who are at high risk for vascular disease and have IFG, IGT, or early diabetes.
- To evaluate the effects of combined treatment with highly purified omega-3 PUFAs plus glargine vs. either intervention alone.

2.3.3. Design (Table 3)

- Randomized, phase III, 2×2 factorial, international, multicenter study.
- Patients are randomized to omega-3 PUFAs vs. placebo or glargine vs. standard care.

Table 3. Design of ORIGIN

	Glargine arm	Standard care arm
OMACOR® arm	Glargine + 1 g/day OMACOR® (n ≈ 2500)	1 g/day OMACOR® (n ≈ 2500)
Placebo arm	Glargine + placebo (n ≈ 2500)	Placebo (n ≈ 2500)

2.3.4. Study Medication Dosages

- 1 g/day OMACOR®.
- Glargine as required to achieve fasting plasma glucose ≤5.3 mmol/L with slow, steady dose escalation.

2.3.5. Patients/Participation Criteria

- Patients aged ≥50 years at risk for CVD according to clinical history, microalbuminuria, or specified investigational criteria plus
- IGT (postprandial plasma glucose (PPG) ≥7.8 and <11.1 mM, with fasting plasma glucose (FPG) <7.0 mM)

or

- IFG (FPG ≥6.1 and <7 mM and no diabetes mellitus (PPG must be <11.1 mM))

or

- Early type-2 diabetes (FPG ≥7.0 mM or PPG ≥11.1 mM) or previous diagnosis of diabetes and no drug therapy during preceding 10 weeks or glycated hemoglobin <150% of upper limit of normal for relevant laboratory

or

- Taking one oral antidiabetic drug, with dose stable for at least 10 weeks immediately preceding the study screening visit.

2.3.6. Exclusion Criteria (Partial Listing)

- Type-1 diabetes mellitus or otherwise requiring insulin.
- Severe heart failure (New York Heart Association (NYHA) functional class ≥3).
- Life expectancy <3 years due to non-cardiovascular causes.

2.3.7. Planned Sample Size

- Number per factorial cell (see Table 3): 2,500; total number of patients: 10,000.

2.3.8. Planned Duration of Follow-Up

- 3-5 years (mean 4 years).

2.3.9. Primary End-Points

- Effect of treatment with highly purified omega-3 PUFAs on cardiovascular morbidity/mortality.
- Effect of glargine-mediated normoglycemia on cardiovascular morbidity/mortality.

2.3.10. Secondary End-Points

(1) Effect of treatment with highly purified omega-3 PUFAs on:
- Major vascular events (composite of cardiovascular death, MI, or stroke).
- Composite of sudden unexpected death, non-sudden arrhythmic death, unwitnessed death, or resuscitated cardiac arrest.
- All-cause mortality.

(2) Effect of glargine-mediated normoglycemia on:
- Risk of diabetic microvascular events.
- Rate of progression of IGT or IFG to type-2 diabetes.
- All-cause mortality.

2.3.11. Schedule

- Start date: August 2003.
- Anticipated completion date: 4Q2008.

ClinicalTrials.gov Identifier: NCT00069784.

2.4. GISSI-HF: GISSI Heart Failure Trial

2.4.1. Rationale

- The GISSI-Prevenzione trial showed that omega-3 PUFAs reduce mortality in patients with a recent MI [20]. A post-hoc analysis showed that this survival benefit extended to a subpopulation of patients with left ventricle dysfunction/failure [26]. Several retrospective investigations of the effect of statins in patients with heart failure also indicated lower mortality in this subset of patients.

2.4.2. Objective

- To investigate whether long-term administration of omega-3 PUFAs or rosuvastatin, or the combination of both, is more effective than placebo in the reduction of all-cause mortality, or all-cause mortality or hospitalizations for any reason in patients with heart failure maintained on best recommended therapies [27].

2.4.3. Design (Figure 1)

- Randomized, double-blind, placebo-controlled, comparator-controlled, multicenter study with two randomizations: first randomization omega-3 PUFAs or placebo (n≈7000); and then second randomization rosuvastatin or placebo (n ≈ 5250).
- Event-driven trial: will continue either until at least 1252 deaths have been recorded in both stages of the randomization or a reduction in all-cause mortality breaches pre-specified stopping boundaries.

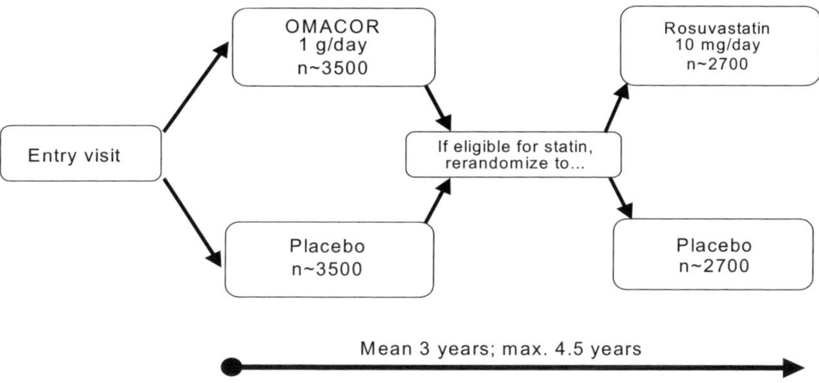

Figure 1. Design of GISSI-HF.

2.4.4. Study Medication Dosages

- 1 g/day OMACOR®.
- 10 mg/day rosuvastatin.
- Matching placebos.

2.4.5. Patients/Participation Criteria*

- Patients with heart failure (NYHA grades II-IV).
- No age requirements/restrictions.

*   Common inclusion conditions for both stages of randomization (see Figure 1).

2.4.6. Planned Sample Size

- Total number of patients for first randomization (see Figure 1): 7,000.
- Total number of patients for second randomization (see Figure 1): 5,250.

2.4.7. Primary End-Points

- All-cause mortality**.
- All-cause mortality or cardiovascular hospitalizations***.

Reductions of **15% and ***20% are considered the minimum clinically relevant outcomes.

2.4.8. Secondary End-Points

- Cardiovascular mortality.
- Cardiovascular mortality or all-cause hospitalizations.
- Sudden cardiac death.
- Hospitalizations for: any reason; cardiovascular reasons; congestive heart failure.
- MI.
- Stroke.

2.4.9. Other Analyses

Multiple pre-specified subgroup analyses of treatment effects to be undertaken, including:
- Age (above/below the median value).
- Left ventricular function (ejection fraction >40% vs. ≤40%).
- Etiology (ischemic vs. non-ischemic).
- Functional capacity (NYHA class II vs. class III-IV).
- Diabetes (yes vs. no).
- Baseline total cholesterol levels (above/below the median value).

2.4.10. Planned Duration of Follow-Up

- Mean 3 years; maximum 4.5 years.

2.4.11. Other

- Study details and updates available at www.GISSI.org.

2.4.12. Schedule

- Recruitment completed September 2005.
- Follow-up in both stages of the randomization to be continued (subject to maximum follow-up 4.5 years) until requisite number of primary end-point events has been accrued.

2.5. GISSI-RP: GISSI Risk and Prevention trial

2.5.1. Rationale

- The results of large trials in cardiovascular prevention conducted over the past decade have stimulated an evolution of cardiovascular risk management. However, there is substantial uncertainty about how successfully these measures are transferred into routine practice, and their overall impact. Although there is now ample evidence in favor of the intensive treatment of patients at high cardiovascular risk [14,23,28-35], surveys of current practice repeatedly report a dissociation between 'recommended' treatment strategies and reality.

2.5.2. Objectives

- To evaluate the efficacy of highly purified omega-3 PUFAs, added to standard conventional measures, in reducing the incidence of cardiovascular events, both fatal and non-fatal, in a population defined as being at high risk by participating general practitioners.
- To evaluate the practicability and effectiveness of the interventions undertaken *(note: this assessment is not limited to the study medication)*.

2.5.3. Design (Figure 2)

- Randomized, placebo-controlled, multicenter study.
- Patients randomized to highly purified omega-3 PUFAs or placebo.

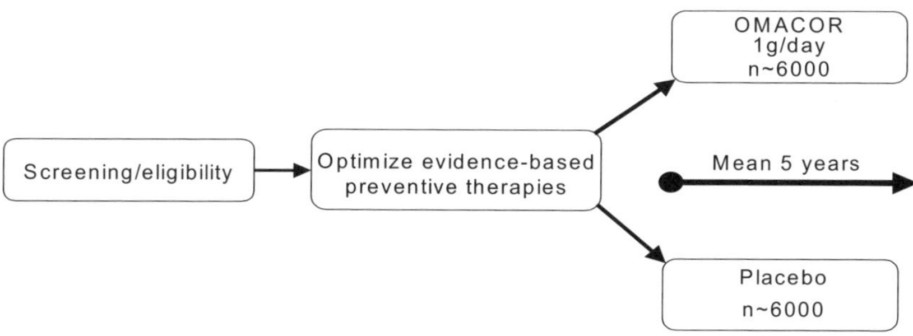

Figure 2. Design of GISSI-RP.

2.5.4. Study Medication Dosages

- 1 g/day OMACOR®.
- Matching placebo.

2.5.5. Patients/Participation Criteria

Patients deemed to be at high cardiovascular risk by the participating general practitioner on the basis of:
- Previous cardio- or cerebrovascular events.
- Presence of risk factors and estimated high 10-year risk for cardio- or cerebrovascular disease.

2.5.6. Exclusion Criteria

- Conditions (e.g. cancer) with unfavorable short-term prognosis.
- Patients unlikely to comply with long-term therapy.

2.5.7. Planned Sample Size

- Total number of patients: 12,000.
- Each participating physician should recruit a minimum of 20 patients (physician network anticipated to be 500-600).

2.5.8. Planned Duration of Follow-Up

- 5 years.

2.5.9. Pre-specified End-Points

- All-cause mortality and non-fatal MI or non-fatal stroke.
- Major cardiovascular events (cardiovascular death, and non-fatal MI or non-fatal stroke).
- Coronary-related mortality.
- Sudden death.

2.5.10. Other

- Statistical methods are predicated on a population of ≈12,000 patients providing power to demonstrate: 15% reduction in total death + non-fatal MI + non-fatal stroke; 20% reduction in cardiovascular death + non-fatal MI + stroke; 30% reduction in cardiovascular death; and 40% reduction in sudden death.

2.5.11. Schedule

- Study started: 2004.

2.6. Omega-3 PUFAs to Prevent Atrial Fibrillation after Cardiovascular Surgery

2.6.1. Rationale

- Atrial fibrillation (AF) is a common complication of cardiothoracic surgery, occurring in up to 4 in 10 patients after CABG and in more than half of patients undergoing CABG plus valvular heart surgery. Postoperative AF does not routinely have long-term sequelae, but the potential for a range of complications (including thromboembolic events) makes it an important and potentially avoidable source of expenditure related to CABG. An intervention that would reduce the incidence of postoperative AF should result in fewer clinical complications and worthwhile cost savings.
- Supplementation with highly purified omega-3 PUFAs has been shown to substantially lower the incidence of sudden death, cardiovascular mortality, and all-cause mortality in post-MI patients [14,36] and meta-analyses of cohort studies support the view that highly purified omega-3 PUFAs reduce cardiovascular risk [37,38]. A cellular basis for a possible role of omega-3 PUFAs in the termination of AF via changes in membrane fluidity has been proposed [39].

2.6.2. Objectives

- To investigate whether pre-treatment with omega-3 PUFAs decreases the incidence of AF in patients undergoing CABG surgery.
- The primary hypothesis is that OMACOR® will significantly reduce the incidence of postoperative AF (vs. placebo).
- The secondary hypothesis is that the length of hospital stay after surgery will be reduced in the patients treated with OMACOR® (vs. placebo).

2.6.3. Design

- Randomized, placebo-controlled, double-blind, prospective study.
- Patients will be randomized to OMACOR® 1 g/day or placebo 3 months before elective CABG.

2.6.4. Study Medication Dosages

- 1 g/day OMACOR®.
- Matching placebo.

2.6.5. Planned Sample Size

- From the assumption that the event rate in the placebo group is 50% and that in the OMACOR® group is 30%, a study with 100 patients/group will have 80% power to detect a difference between the study treatments (two-tailed alpha = 0.05).

2.6.6. Patients/Participation Criteria

- Men or women aged >65 years scheduled to undergo elective CABG.

2.6.7. Exclusion Criteria

- NYHA heart failure class IV.
- Chronic AF or flutter.
- Current use of implantable cardiac defibrillator or implantable pacemakers.
- Second- or third-degree atrioventricular block.
- Significant thyroid, pulmonary, or hepatic disease.
- Significant clotting disorders or impairment of renal function.
- Contraindications to study medication.

2.6.8. Planned Duration of Follow-Up

- 30 days or hospital discharge, whichever occurs later.

2.6.9. Primary End-Point

- Effect (if any) of OMACOR® treatment on the development of AF within 30 days of cardiothoracic surgery.

2.6.10. Secondary End-Point

- Effect (if any) of OMACOR® treatment on the length of postoperative hospital stay.

2.6.11. Schedule

- Study start: August 2005.

2.7. OPACH: Prevention of Cardiovascular Events in Patients Undergoing Chronic Hemodialysis

2.7.1. Rationale

- CVD is widespread among patients with end-stage renal disease (ESRD) and is estimated to account for at least half of the deaths in this high-risk population. The overall risk profile of ESRD patients means, however, that they are often excluded from clinical trials investigating secondary prevention of cardiac events, so there is little reliable information about what measures might be of benefit. There is evidence from the GISSI-Prevenzione study that omega-3 PUFAs reduce mortality in patients with CVD [14], but there have been no well-designed studies of the effects (if any) of omega-3 PUFAs in hemodialysis patients with CVD.

2.7.2. Objective

- To examine the effects of treatment with highly purified omega-3 PUFAs on the incidence of cardiovascular events and cardiovascular deaths in ESRD patients who have documented CVD and who are undergoing chronic dialysis.

2.7.3. Design (Figure 3)

- Randomized, placebo-controlled, double-blind, parallel-group, multicenter study.
- Patients are randomized to OMACOR® or placebo in addition to standard care.

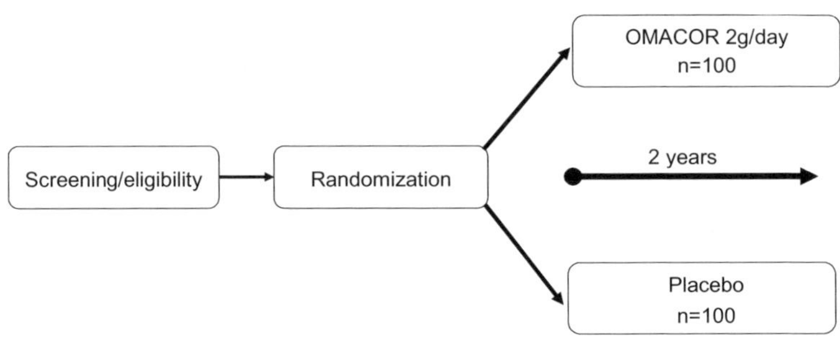

Figure 3. Design of OPACH.

2.7.4. Study Medication Dosages*

- 2 g/day OMACOR®.
- Matching placebos.

* Other medications will be continued or introduced as required based on clinical considerations of patient welfare.

2.7.5. Patients/Participation Criteria

- Men or women aged >18 years on hemodialysis for ≥6 months *and* at least one of:
- Angina pectoris diagnosed by specified clinical criteria.
- Previous acute MI diagnosed by specified clinical criteria.
- Previous PTCA/CABG or angiographically proven coronary atherosclerosis.
- Previous TIA diagnosed by specified clinical criteria.
- Previous stroke, defined as sudden focal neurological symptoms persisting for >24 hours.
- Clinical diagnosis of peripheral vascular disease diagnosed by specified criteria.

2.7.6. Exclusion Criteria (Partial Listing)

- Active malignant disease, except basal cell carcinoma or spinocellular carcinoma.
- Peritoneal dialysis.

2.7.7. Planned Sample Size

- 100 patients per arm; total number of patients: 200.

2.7.8. Planned Duration of Follow-Up

- 2 years.

2.7.9. Primary End-Points**

- Cardiovascular event (angina, MI, stroke, TIA, or new symptoms of peripheral vascular disease) or death.

** Patients who experience a primary end-point will be withdrawn from the study. Time to primary end-point event will be recorded as part of the study analysis.

2.7.10. Secondary End-Points

- Effect on heart rate variability.
- Thrombosis or stenosis of the dialysis graft.

2.7.11. Schedule

- Start date: November 2002.
- Anticipated completion date: February 2005.

2.8. OCEAN: Effect of Omega-3 PUFAs on Plaque Stability in Patients Awaiting Endarterectomy

2.8.1. Rationale

- Omega-3 PUFAs have been shown to protect against death from CVD, in particular sudden death [14,26]. One hypothesis advanced to explain this effect is that incorporation of omega-3 PUFAs into atherosclerotic plaques might stabilize them by reducing the infiltration of inflammatory cells.

2.8.2. Objective

- To investigate whether OMACOR® has potentially beneficial effects on the stability of plaques in the carotid arteries.

2.8.3. Design (Figure 4)

- Randomized, placebo-controlled, double-blind, parallel-group, multicenter study.
- Patients are randomized to OMACOR® or placebo.

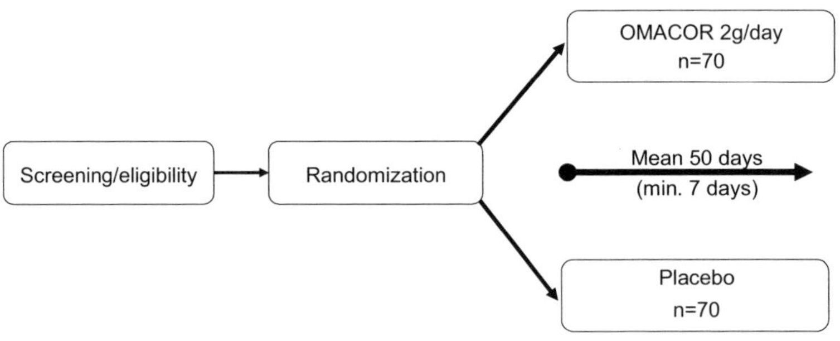

Figure 4. Design of OCEAN.

2.8.4. Study Medication Dosages

- 2 g/day OMACOR®.
- Matching placebos.

2.8.5. Patients/Participation Criteria

- Men or women aged >18 years awaiting carotid endarterectomy.

2.8.6. Exclusion Criteria

- Endarterectomy due within 7 days.
- Using fish oil or evening primrose oil supplements.
- >2 oily fish meals/week.

2.8.7. Planned Sample Size

- 70 patients per arm; total number of patients: 140.

2.8.8. Planned Duration of Follow-Up

- Mean 50 days (minimum 7 days, ending 1 day before surgery).

2.8.9. Primary End-Point

- Content of omega-3 fatty acids in carotid plaques after treatment.

2.8.10. Secondary End-Points

Investigation of:
- Morphology of carotid plaques.
- Macrophage and activated T-lymphocyte infiltration in carotid plaques.
- Levels of matrix metalloproteinase, cytokine and peroxisome proliferator-activated receptor (PPAR) isoform proteins and mRNA in carotid plaques.
- Quantity of omega-3 fatty acids in plasma phospholipids.

2.8.11. Laboratory Measurements

- Determination of eicosapentaenoic acid (EPA) and docosahexaenoic acid (DHA) in plaques.

2.8.12. Other

- This study supplements earlier research by the same investigators in which it was shown that atherosclerotic plaques incorporated omega-3 PUFAs from supplements and that this incorporation induced morphological changes thought likely to enhance plaque stability. No comparable effect was observed after supplementation with omega-6 PUFAs (sunflower oil) [40].

2.8.13. Schedule

- Start date: November 2003.
- Status: patient recruitment finalized.

3. Ongoing Controlled Trials of OMACOR® 4 g/day

3.1. OMACOR® in IgA Nephropathy

3.1.1. Rationale

- IgA nephropathy is the most common cause of primary glomerulonephritis. The primary cause of the disease is unknown and its molecular mechanisms have not been fully elucidated. The rate of progression is highly variable and the condition may be benign; however, a high proportion of patients with this condition (up to 40%) progress to ESRD. The disease may occur at any age, including in childhood, and often affects young adults. It may therefore impose a particularly severe burden of illness. IgA nephropathy is estimated to affect 1% of many populations [41].
- Some of the best available evidence of treatment benefit has been accrued with omega-3 PUFA therapy. Long-term use of OMACOR® at a daily dose of 4 g has been shown to reduce the increase in serum creatinine and the development of ESRD in patients with IgA nephropathy [42]. More recently, it has been demonstrated in a RCT that the maximum dose necessary to derive full therapeutic benefit from OMACOR® is 4 g/day [43]; it has been suggested that lower doses of omega-3 PUFAs may be effective but the database in support of this suggestion is currently small [44].
- Preservation of renal function has not been demonstrated in controlled trials of angiotensin-converting enzyme (ACE) inhibitors in IgA nephropathy but these drugs are widely used to control hypertension in this situation and have been shown to relieve proteinuria [41].
- Corticosteroids preserve renal function in IgA nephropathy but high doses appear to be necessary [45,46] and the long-term use of such a regimen brings risks of its own [41].
- Mycophenolate mofetil (MMF) is an immunosuppressant that has been evaluated for the management of IgA nephropathy. Results to date have been mixed, with evidence of benefit on proteinuria and lipid profile but none on renal function in patients with established disease [47-50].

3.1.2. Objectives

- To evaluate the effect of adding MMF to existing therapy of OMACOR® and lisinopril.
- To examine the effect of 2.25 years of continuous therapy with OMACOR® and lisinopril.

3.1.3. Design (Figure 5)

- Randomized, placebo-controlled, double-blind, multicenter study.
- Patients receive OMACOR® plus lisinopril, followed after 3 months by MMF or placebo for 1 year (losartan may be substituted for lisinopril if necessary).

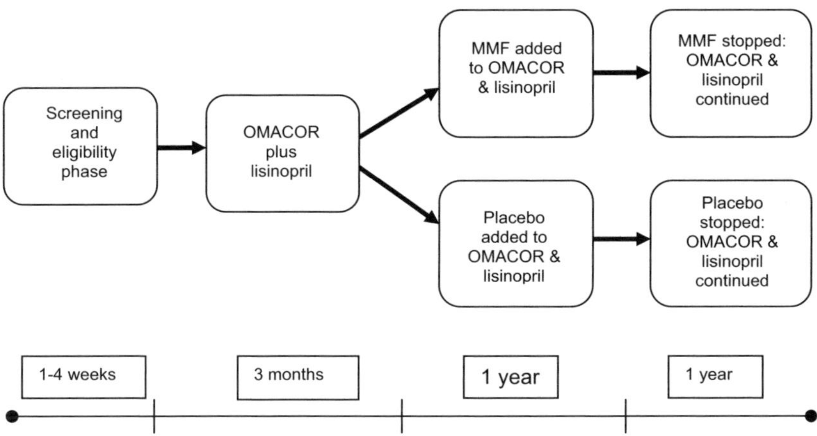

Figure 5. Design of study.

3.1.4. Study Medication Dosages

- 4 g/day OMACOR® if body surface area ≥ 1 m^2. Dose adjusted for patients with lower body surface area.
- 5-20 mg/day lisinopril according to a weight-adjusted schedule. Subject to tolerance, dose is doubled after 1 month, with option for further doubling after another 4 weeks if necessary to control blood pressure.
- 25-35 mg/kg/day MMF to a maximum of 1 g b.i.d. according to a weight-adjusted schedule, or matching placebo.

3.1.5. Planned Sample Size

- 100 patients (from an initial screening cohort of 200).
- Sample size/power calculations assume (a) that OMACOR® or lisinopril will reduce urinary protein:creatinine ratio from 1.90 to 1.20 during the initial 3 months and thereafter maintain it at that level, and (b) that introduction of MMF will further reduce the mean protein:creatinine ratio to 0.50.

3.1.6. Patients/Participation Criteria

- Men or women aged >7 years and <70 years.
- Renal biopsy diagnostic for IgA neuropathy (enrollment not dependent on interval between biopsy and time of study entry).
- Urine protein:creatinine ratio ≥ 0.6 for males and ≥ 0.8 for females prior to randomization.
- Negative pregnancy test 1 week prior to starting lisinopril for females of childbearing potential, repeated <1 week before starting MMF or placebo.
- Estimated glomerular filtration rate (estGFR) ≥ 40 ml/min/1.73 m^2 at randomization.

3.1.7. Exclusion Criteria (Partial Listing)

- Clinical and histologic evidence of systemic lupus erythematosus or well-documented history of Henoch-Schönlein purpura.
- Cirrhosis, chronic active liver disease, hepatitis B, hepatitis C.
- History of significant gastrointestinal disorder.
- HIV-positive.
- Systemic infection or history of serious infection within 1 month of entry.
- Absolute neutrophil count $<2000/mm^3$ or hematocrit $<28\%$.
- estGFR <40 ml/min/1.73 m^2 at time of randomization (decline below that level during treatment with MMF or placebo acceptable provided rate before randomization is $\geq 60\%$ of the pre-entry value).
- Other major organ system disease or malignancy except skin cancer fully excised >5 years prior to entry.

3.1.8. Planned Duration of Follow-Up

- 2 years from initiation of MMF therapy, including 12 months of follow-up after cessation of MMF therapy. Estimated total duration of study: 4-5 years.

3.1.9. Primary End-points

- Change from baseline in urinary protein:creatinine ratio. Change in the ratio will be examined and quantified by (a) Kaplan-Meier time-to-event analysis and (b) rate of change in the ratio.

3.1.10. Secondary End-Points

- Change in estGFR during the study. (It is recognized that there is only limited likelihood of detecting a change in this outcome in a relatively short-term study.)

3.1.11. Other

- A separate 1-year study to evaluate the effect of MMF plus ACE-inhibitor therapy in early IgA nephropathy has been proposed [57].

3.1.12. Schedule

- Study start: March 2005.
- Recruitment of patients: ongoing.
- Anticipated completion date: 2008-9.

ISRCTN Identifier: 62574616.

3.2.   OM5: Adjunctive OMACOR® Therapy in Hypertriglyceridemic Subjects Treated with Antara™

3.2.1. Rationale

- Fibrates significantly reduce fasting triglyceride concentrations (by 20-50%) and postprandial triglyceride concentrations and increase the concentration of high-density lipoprotein (HDL) cholesterol (by 10-35%). These agents also promote qualitative changes in the lipoprotein profile that are considered to reduce atherogenic potential [52,53]. These changes in lipid/lipoprotein profile, supplemented by potentially advantageous alterations in various haemostatic and inflammatory markers, are thought to contribute to the anti-atherogenic and cardioprotective effects of fibrate therapy [54,55]. Fenofibrate is an exemplar of the fibrate class and has been the object of several clinical trials, notably among patients with hypertriglyceridemia or diabetes [56,57]. The drug has relatively poor bioavailability. Antara™, a new formulation of fenofibrate (as micronized granules) designed to address this limitation of fenofibrate, will be examined in this study.
- Omega-3 PUFAs also lower plasma triglyceride levels. An examination of 65 clinical trials indicated that supplementation with ≈3-4 g/day of omega-3 PUFAs lowered triglyceride levels by 25-30% vs. controls [58]. The ability of omega-3 PUFAs to lower triglyceride concentrations seems to be proportional to the severity of baseline hypertriglyceridemia. OMACOR®, at doses of 3-4 g/day, demonstrated considerable triglyceride-lowering efficacy in patients with familial combined hyperlipidemia [59] and in those with hypertriglyceridemia, whether as monotherapy [60] or in combination with a statin [24].

3.2.2. Objectives

- To determine whether the combination of OMACOR® plus micronized fenofibrate is more effective for the management of hypertriglyceridemia than micronized fenofibrate alone.
- To compare the safety profile and tolerability of OMACOR® plus micronized fenofibrate with those of micronized fenofibrate alone in patients with hypertriglyceridemia.

3.2.3. Design

- Randomized, double-blind, placebo-controlled, parallel-group study.
- Patients receive micronized fenofibrate plus OMACOR® or placebo.

3.2.4. Study Medication Dosages

- Micronized fenofibrate 130 mg/day *plus*:
- 4 g/day OMACOR®

or

- placebo.

3.2.5. Planned Sample Size

- 75 patients per treatment arm; total number of patients: 150.

3.2.6. Patients/Participation Criteria

- Men or women aged 18-79 years, inclusive.
- Fasting triglyceride levels $\geq$500 mg/dl and <1000 mg/dl (5.7-11.3 mmol/l) (average of the values at the two screening visits at weeks -2 and -1).
- Body-mass index $\geq$25 kg/m^2 and $\leq$40 kg/m^2 at visit 1.
- All patients comply with the US National Cholesterol Education Program Therapeutic Lifestyle Change diet during the 6-week run-in period.

3.2.7. Exclusion Criteria (Partial Listing)

- Any non-study-related use of: omega-3 PUFA supplements, or niacin or its analogs at doses of >400 mg/day during run-in phase.
- Any non-study-related use of any lipid-altering drugs, including statins, bile acid sequestrants, cholesterol absorption inhibitors, or fibrates during either run-in or active phases of the study.
- Lipoprotein lipase impairment or apo C-2 deficiency or type-III hyperlipidemia.
- History of pancreatitis.
- Type-1 diabetes or poorly controlled diabetes mellitus.
- Use of isotretinoin or warfarin.

3.2.8. Planned Duration of Follow-Up

- 6-week run-in followed by 8 weeks of active therapy.

3.2.9. Primary End-Points

- Percent change in plasma triglycerides from baseline (average of weeks -2, -1, and 0) to the end of double-blind treatment (average of weeks 6 and 8).

3.2.10. Secondary End-Points

- Percent changes from baseline to the end of double-blind treatment for: total cholesterol; very-LDL cholesterol; LDL cholesterol; HDL cholesterol; total cholesterol:HDL ratio; non-HDL cholesterol; apolipoprotein A1; and apolipoprotein B.

3.2.11. Other

- All participants who complete the initial double-blind study will be eligible for an open-label extension phase. Participants in that phase will receive open-label micronized fenofibrate at 130 mg/day plus open-label OMACOR® at 4 g/day for a further 8 weeks.

3.2.12. Schedule

- Study start: November 2005.
- Recruitment of patients: ongoing.
- Anticipated completion date: June 2006.

ClinicalTrials.gov Identifier: NCT00246636.

3.3. OM6: Combined OMACOR® and Simvastatin Therapy in Hypertriglyceridemic Subjects

3.3.1. Rationale

- Currently, the most commonly used lipid-altering drugs are statins. These drugs substantially reduce LDL cholesterol and have been shown to be consistently highly effective in reducing the risk of CHD [21], but produce less expansive reductions in triglyceride unless there is marked baseline hypertriglyceridemia [61,62].
- Statin therapy may therefore be an incomplete response to lipid-mediated CHD risk because elevated triglyceride levels have been identified as an independent risk factor for CHD [63-65].
- A review of 65 clinical trials showed that supplementation with an average of 3-4 g/day of omega-3 PUFAs lowered triglyceride levels by 25-30% vs. controls [58]. Combination of OMACOR® with a statin thus has potential to augment the relatively modest effect of the statin alone on plasma triglyceride levels. The present trial will extend the investigation of OMACOR® to less severe hypertriglyceridemia than has previously been evaluated in clinical trials [24] and assess the efficacy of OMACOR® when taken in combination with a statin.

3.3.2. Objectives

- To assess the efficacy of OMACOR® 4 g/day combined with simvastatin 40 mg/day for lowering non-HDL cholesterol levels in patients with persistent hypertriglyceridemia despite statin therapy.
- To assess the safety of OMACOR® 4 g/day combined with simvastatin 40 mg/day.

3.3.3. Design

- Randomized, double-blind, placebo-controlled, parallel study.
- Double-blind OMACOR® vs. placebo.
- Open-label simvastatin treatment.

3.3.4. Study Medication Dosage

- 4 g/day OMACOR®.
- 40 mg/day simvastatin.

3.3.5. Planned Sample Size

- 111 patients in each treatment group; total number of patients: 222.

3.3.6. Patients/Participation Criteria

- Men and women aged 18-79 years, inclusive.
- Current statin use for control of LDL cholesterol at visit 1 (with dose stable for at least 8 weeks).
- Fasting triglyceride level $\geq$200 mg/dl and <500 mg/dl (2.3-5.6 mmol/l) (average of weeks -2 and -1).
- Patient's average LDL cholesterol concentration at or below the relevant goal (as described in the provisions of the US National Cholesterol Education Program Adult Treatment Panel III) at weeks -2 and -1 (in recognition of variability of lipid levels, participants within 10% of LDL goal will be considered eligible).

3.3.7. Exclusion Criteria (Partial Listing)

- Any use of non-study-related lipid-altering drugs after first clinical visit.
- Lipoprotein lipase impairment or apo C-2 deficiency or type-III hyperlipidemia.
- Unexplained muscle pain or weakness.
- History of pancreatitis.
- Poorly controlled diabetes, or receiving insulin therapy.
- Use of warfarin.

3.3.8. Planned Duration of Follow-Up

- 8-week lead-in period; 8-week treatment period.

3.3.9. Primary End-Point

- Percent change in non-HDL cholesterol from baseline.

3.3.10. Secondary End-Points

- Percent change from baseline in: total cholesterol; very-LDL cholesterol; LDL cholesterol; HDL cholesterol; total cholesterol:HDL ratio; non-HDL cholesterol; apolipoprotein A1; and apolipoprotein B.

3.3.11. Schedule

- Study start: May 2005.
- Recruitment of patients: ongoing.
- Anticipated completion date: 2006.

ClinicalTrials.gov Identifier: NCT00246701.

References

[1]   R.B. Haynes, C.D. Mulrow, E.J. Huth *et al.* More informative abstracts revisited. *Ann. Intern. Med.* **113** (1990) 69-76.

[2]   D.L. Sackett, W.M. Rosenberg, J.A. Gray *et al.* Evidence based medicine: what it is and what it isn't. *BMJ* **312** (1996) 71-72.

[3]   C. Young and R. Horton. Putting clinical trials into context. *Lancet* **366** (2005) 107-108.

[4]   A.L. Cochrane. Foreword. In: I. Chalmers, M. Enkin, M.J.N.C. Keirse (Eds): *Effective care in pregnancy and childbirth.* Oxford, UK: Oxford University Press (1989).

[5]   A. Stang, H.W. Hense, K.H. Jockel *et al.* Is it always unethical to use a placebo in a clinical trial? *PLoS Med.* **2** (2005) e72.

[6]   J. Olsson, D. Terris, M. Elg *et al.* The one-person randomized controlled trial. *Qual. Manag. Health Care* **14** (2005) 206-216.

[7]   G. Block, T. Block, P. Wakimoto *et al.* Demonstration of an e-mailed worksite nutrition intervention program. *Prev. Chronic Dis.* **1** (2004) A06.

[8]   D. Dreyfuss. Beyond randomized, controlled trials. *Curr. Opin. Crit. Care* **10** (2004) 574-578.

[9]   V.M. Montori. Evidence-based endocrinology: how far have we come? *Treat Endocrinol.* **3** (2004) 1-10.

[10]   J. Grossman and F.J. Mackenzie. The randomized controlled trial: gold standard, or merely standard? *Perspect. Biol. Med.* **48** (2005) 516-534.

[11]   B. Druss. Evidence based medicine: does it make a difference? Use wisely. *BMJ* **330** (2005) 92.

[12]   A. Kotaska. Inappropriate use of randomised trials to evaluate complex phenomena: case study of vaginal breech delivery. *BMJ* **329** (2004) 1039-1042.

[13]   I. Boutron, P. Ravaud, B. Giraudeau. Inappropriateness of randomised trials for complex phenomena: single trial is never enough evidence to base decisions on. *BMJ* **330** (2005) 94.

[14]   GISSI-Prevenzione Investigators. Dietary supplementation with n-3 polyunsaturated fatty acids and vitamin E after myocardial infarction: results of the GISSI-Prevenzione trial. Gruppo Italiano per lo Studio della Sopravvivenza nell'Infarto miocardico. *Lancet* **354** (1999) 447-455.

[15]   Heart Protection Study Collaborative Group. MRC/BHF Heart Protection Study of antioxidant vitamin supplementation in 20,536 high-risk individuals: a randomised placebo-controlled trial. *Lancet* **360** (2002) 23-33.

[16]   S. Yusuf, G. Dagenais, J. Pogue *et al.* Vitamin E supplementation and cardiovascular events in high-risk patients. The Heart Outcomes Prevention Evaluation Study Investigators. *N. Engl. J. Med.* **342** (2000) 154-160.

[17]   I.M. Lee, N.R. Cook, J.M. Gaziano *et al.* Vitamin E in the primary prevention of cardiovascular disease and cancer: the Women's Health Study: a randomized controlled trial. *JAMA* **294** (2005) 56-65.

[18]   S. Devaraj and I. Jialal. Failure of vitamin E in clinical trials: is gamma-tocopherol the answer? *Nutr. Rev.* **63** (2005) 290-293.

[19]   K.H. Bonaa, I. Njolstad, P.M. Ueland *et al.* NORVIT Trial Investigators. Homocysteine lowering and cardiovascular events after acute myocardial infarction. *N. Engl. J. Med.* **354** (2006) 1578-1588.

[20]   M.R. Olthof, T. van Vliet, P. Verhoef *et al.* Effect of homocysteine-lowering nutrients on blood lipids: results from four randomised, placebo-controlled studies in healthy humans. *PLoS Med.* **2** (2005) e135.

[21]   R. Clarke. Homocysteine-lowering trials for prevention of heart disease and stroke. *Semin. Vasc. Med.* **5** (2005) 215-222.

[22]   H. King, R.E. Aubert, W.H. Herman. Global burden of diabetes 1995-2025: prevalence, numerical estimates, and projections. *Diabetes Care* **21** (1998) 1414-1431.

[23]   C. Baigent, A. Keech, P.M. Kearney *et al.* Efficacy and safety of cholesterol-lowering treatment: prospective meta-analysis of data from 90,056 participants in 14 randomised trials of statins. *Lancet* **366** (2005) 1267-1278.

[24]   P.N. Durrington, D. Bhatnagar, M.I. Mackness *et al.* An omega-3 polyunsaturated fatty acid concentrate administered for one year decreased triglycerides in simvastatin treated patients with coronary heart disease and persisting hypertriglyceridaemia. *Heart* **85** (2001) 544-548.

[25]   S. Wild, G. Roglic, A. Green *et al.* Global prevalence of diabetes: estimates for the year 2000 and projections for 2030. *Diabetes Care* **27** (2004) 1047-1053.

[26]   A. Macchia, G. Levantesi, M.G. Franzosi *et al.* Left ventricular systolic dysfunction, total mortality, and sudden death in patients with myocardial infarction treated with n-3 polyunsaturated fatty acids. *Eur. J. Heart Fail.* **7** (2005) 904-909.

[27]   L. Tavazzi, G. Tognoni, M.G. Franzosi *et al*. Rationale and design of the GISSI heart failure trial: a large trial to assess the effects of n-3 polyunsaturated fatty acids and rosuvastatin in symptomatic congestive heart failure. *Eur. J. Heart Fail.* **6** (2004) 635-641.

[28]   B. Dahlof, P.S. Sever, N.R. Poulter *et al*. Prevention of cardiovascular events with an antihypertensive regimen of amlodipine adding perindopril as required versus atenolol adding bendroflumethiazide as required, in the Anglo-Scandinavian Cardiac Outcomes Trial-Blood Pressure Lowering Arm (ASCOT-BPLA): a multicentre randomised controlled trial. *Lancet* **366** (2005) 895-906.

[29]   H.M. Colhoun, D.J. Betteridge, P.N. Durrington *et al*. Primary prevention of cardiovascular disease with atorvastatin in type 2 diabetes in the Collaborative Atorvastatin Diabetes Study (CARDS): multicentre randomised placebo-controlled trial. *Lancet* **364** (2004) 685-696.

[30]   S. Yusuf, P. Sleight, J. Pogue *et al*. Effects of an angiotensin-converting-enzyme inhibitor, ramipril, on cardiovascular events in high-risk patients. The Heart Outcomes Prevention Evaluation Study Investigators. *N. Engl. J. Med.* **342** (2000) 145-153.

[31]   J. Schrader, S. Luders, A. Kulschewski *et al*. Morbidity and mortality after stroke, eprosartan compared with nitrendipine for secondary prevention: principal results of a prospective randomized controlled study (MOSES). *Stroke* **36** (2005) 1218-1226.

[32]   F. Turnbull and the Blood Pressure Lowering Treatment Trialists' Collaboration. Effects of different blood-pressure-lowering regimens on major cardiovascular events: results of prospectively-designed overviews of randomised trials. *Lancet* **362** (2003) 1527-1535.

[33]   J.L. Chiasson, R.G. Josse, R. Gomis *et al*. Acarbose treatment and the risk of cardiovascular disease and hypertension in patients with impaired glucose tolerance: the STOP-NIDDM trial. *JAMA* **290** (2003) 486-494.

[34]   W. Bestermann, M.C. Houston, J. Basile *et al*. Addressing the global cardiovascular risk of hypertension, dyslipidemia, diabetes mellitus, and the metabolic syndrome in the southeastern United States, part II: treatment recommendations for management of the global cardiovascular risk of hypertension, dyslipidemia, diabetes mellitus, and the metabolic syndrome. *Am. J. Med. Sci.* **329** (2005) 292-305.

[35]   R. Ratner, R. Goldberg, S. Haffner *et al*. Impact of intensive lifestyle and metformin therapy on cardiovascular disease risk factors in the diabetes prevention program. *Diabetes Care* **28** (2005) 888-894.

[36]   R. Marchioli, F. Barzi, E. Bomba *et al*. Early protection against sudden death by n-3 polyunsaturated fatty acids after myocardial infarction: time-course analysis of the results of the Gruppo Italiano per lo Studio della Sopravvivenza nell'Infarto Miocardico (GISSI)-Prevenzione. *Circulation* **105** (2002) 1897-1903.

[37]   H.C. Bucher, P. Hengstler, C. Schindler *et al*. N-3 polyunsaturated fatty acids in coronary heart disease: a meta-analysis of randomized controlled trials. *Am. J. Med.* **112** (2002) 298-304.

[38]   K. He, Y. Song, M.L. Daviglus *et al*. Accumulated evidence on fish consumption and coronary heart disease mortality: a meta-analysis of cohort studies. *Circulation* **109** (2004) 2705-2711.

[39]   A. Jahangiri, W.R. Leifert, G.S. Patten *et al*. Termination of asynchronous contractile activity in rat atrial myocytes by n-3 polyunsaturated fatty acids. *Mol. Cell. Biochem.* **206** (2000) 33-41.

[40]   F. Thies, J.M. Garry, P. Yaqoob *et al*. Association of n-3 polyunsaturated fatty acids with stability of atherosclerotic plaques: a randomised controlled trial. *Lancet* **361** (2003) 477-485.

[41]   J.V. Donadio and J.P. Grande. IgA nephropathy. *N. Engl. J. Med.* **347** (2002) 738-748.

[42]   J.V. Donadio Jr, J.P. Grande, E.J. Bergstralh *et al*. The long-term outcome of patients with IgA nephropathy treated with fish oil in a controlled trial. Mayo Nephrology Collaborative Group. *J. Am. Soc. Nephrol.* **10** (1999) 1772-1777.

[43]   J.V. Donadio Jr, T.S. Larson, E.J. Bergstralh *et al*. A randomized trial of high-dose compared with low-dose omega-3 fatty acids in severe IgA nephropathy. *J. Am. Soc. Nephrol.* **12** (2001) 791-799.

[44]   E. Alexopoulos, M. Stangou, A. Pantzaki *et al*. Treatment of severe IgA nephropathy with omega-3 fatty acids: the effect of a "very low dose" regimen. *Ren. Fail.* **26** (2004) 453-459.

[45]   C. Pozzi, P.G. Bolasco, G.B. Fogazzi *et al*. Corticosteroids in IgA nephropathy: a randomised controlled trial. *Lancet* **353** (1999) 883-887.

[46]   R. Katafuchi, K. Ikeda, T. Mizumasa *et al*. Controlled, prospective trial of steroid treatment in IgA nephropathy: a limitation of low-dose prednisolone therapy. *Am. J. Kidney Dis.* **41** (2003) 972-983.

[47]   X. Chen, P. Chen, G. Cai *et al*. A randomized control trial of mycophenolate mofeil treatment in severe IgA nephropathy. *Zhonghua Yi Xue Za Zhi* **82** (2002) 796-801 (*in Chinese*).

[48]   S. Tang, J.C.K. Leung, A.W.C. Tang *et al*. A prospective, randomized, case-controlled study on the efficacy of mycophenolate mofetil (MMF) for IgA nephropathy (IgAN) patients with persistent proteinuria despite angiotensin blockade. *J. Am. Soc. Nephrol.* **14** (2003) 752A-753A.

[49]　B.D. Maes, R. Oyen, K. Claes *et al.* Mycophenolate mofetil in IgA nephropathy: results of a 3-year prospective placebo-controlled randomized study. *Kidney Int.* **65** (2004) 1842-1849.

[50]　G. Frisch, J. Lin, J. Rosenstock *et al.* Mycophenolate mofetil (MMF) vs placebo in patients with moderately advanced IgA nephropathy: a double-blind randomized controlled trial. *Nephrol. Dial. Transplant.* **20** (2005) 2139-2145.

[51]　A. Dal Canton, A. Amore, G. Barbano *et al.* One-year angiotensin-converting enzyme inhibition plus mycophenolate mofetil immunosuppression in the course of early IgA nephropathy: a multicenter, randomised, controlled study. *J. Nephrol.* **18** (2005) 136-140.

[52]　K. Ikewaki, J. Tohyama, Y. Nakata *et al.* Fenofibrate effectively reduces remnants, and small dense LDL, and increases HDL particle number in hypertriglyceridemic men - a nuclear magnetic resonance study. *J. Atheroscler. Thromb.* **11** (2004) 278-285.

[53]　K. Winkler, P. Weltzien, I. Friedrich *et al.* Qualitative effect of fenofibrate and quantitative effect of atorvastatin on LDL profile in combined hyperlipidemia with dense LDL. *Exp. Clin. Endocrinol. Diabetes* **112** (2004) 241-247.

[54]　K. Kon Koh, J. Yeal Ahn, S. Hwan Han *et al.* Effects of fenofibrate on lipoproteins, vasomotor function, and serological markers of inflammation, plaque stabilization, and hemostasis. *Atherosclerosis* **174** (2004) 379-383.

[55]　E. Coban and R. Sari. The effect of fenofibrate on the levels of high sensitivity C-reactive protein in dyslipidemic obese patients. *Endocr. Res.* **30** (2004) 343-349.

[56]　G. Derosa, A.E. Cicero, G. Bertone *et al.* Comparison of fluvastatin + fenofibrate combination therapy and fluvastatin monotherapy in the treatment of combined hyperlipidemia, type 2 diabetes mellitus, and coronary heart disease: a 12-month, randomized, double-blind, controlled trial. *Clin. Ther.* **26** (2004) 1599-1607.

[57]　J.C. Ansquer, C. Foucher, S. Rattier *et al.* Fenofibrate reduces progression to microalbuminuria over 3 years in a placebo-controlled study in type 2 diabetes: results from the Diabetes Atherosclerosis Intervention Study (DAIS). *Am. J. Kidney Dis.* **45** (2005) 485-493.

[58]　W.S. Harris. n-3 fatty acids and serum lipoproteins: human studies. *Am. J. Clin. Nutr.* **65** (1997) 1645S-1654S.

[59]　L. Calabresi, D. Donati, F. Pazzucconi *et al.* Omacor in familial combined hyperlipidemia: effects on lipids and low density lipoprotein subclasses. *Atherosclerosis* **148** (2000) 387-396.

[60]　W.S. Harris, H.N. Ginsberg, N. Arunakul *et al.* Safety and efficacy of Omacor in severe hypertriglyceridemia. *J. Cardiovasc. Risk* **4** (1997) 385-391.

[61]　E.A. Stein, M. Lane, P. Laskarzewski. Comparison of statins in hypertriglyceridemia. *Am. J. Cardiol.* **81** (1998) 66B-69B.

[62]　J. Isaacsohn, D. Hunninghake, H. Schrott *et al.* Effects of simvastatin, an HMG-CoA reductase inhibitor, in patients with hypertriglyceridemia. *Clin. Cardiol.* **26** (2003) 18-24.

[63]　M.H. Criqui, G. Heiss, R. Cohn *et al.* Plasma triglyceride level and mortality from coronary heart disease. *N. Engl. J. Med.* **328** (1993) 1220-1225.

[64]　J.E. Hokanson and M.A. Austin. Plasma triglyceride is a risk factor for cardiovascular disease independent of high-density lipoprotein cholesterol level: a meta-analysis of population-based prospective studies. *J. Cardiovasc. Risk* **3** (1996) 213-219.

[65]　G. Assmann, H. Schulte, H. Funke *et al.* The emergence of triglycerides as a significant independent risk factor in coronary artery disease. *Eur. Heart J.* **19 (Suppl. M)** (1998) M8-M14.

Cardiovascular Benefits of Omega-3 Polyunsaturated Fatty Acids
B. Maisch and R. Oelze (Eds.)
IOS Press, 2006

Author Index